"Art therapist Megu Kitazawa has written a book rich with information and insight which will be wonderful in the training and development of both future art therapists, as well as expanding the mostly Eurocentric literature available for current professionals in the field. *Asian Art Therapists: Navigating Art, Diversity, and Culture* is timely and sorely needed as we all learn to work effectively together in our interdependent world. This book is a true gift to our profession and a must-read for all."

Stephanie Wise, ATR-BC, ATCS, LCAT,
director, Art Therapy Program, Marywood University, USA

"*Asian Art Therapists* is a much-needed book for professionals and multicultural studies. Megu Kitazawa asks important questions about the training and profession of art therapy. Through her thoughtful, self-reflective chapter to a selection of narratives from Asian art therapists this is required reading for all."

Val Sereno, ATR-BC, LCAT,
coordinator of Special Programs and
Projects at the School of Visual Arts, USA

"The first book of its kind, *Asian Art Therapists: Navigating Art, Diversity, and Culture* is a must-read for all therapists and students. Powerful, moving, and illuminating: the voices of the authors inspire meaningful reflection and call to action."

Raquel Chapin Stephenson, PhD, ATR-BC, LCAT,
associate professor, Art Therapy Program Coordinator,
Expressive Therapies Division, Lesley University, USA

"*Asian Art Therapists* invites the reader to join the tremendous and touching journey of self discovery the therapists portrayed here have made, articulating for themselves and their surroundings their racial, ethnic, familial, personal and professional identities. Varied and multi voiced, these narratives tell a tale of loss and gain, of growing clarity and ease that come from learning who you are. Simultaneously, it is an important step in portraying the need and making space for further growth, diversity and inclusiveness in the field of psychotherapy."

Tamar Talmi, MA,
psychologist in private practice in Berlin, Germany

"This book is such a gift. So grateful for each of these art thera-pist's and client's voices as they provide opportunities to reflect on the nuances of cross-cultural work, and how identity impacts our approach to therapy and education."

Shannon Bradley, ATR-BC, LCAT, psychotherapist,
Pratt Instructor and Low Residency Co-coordinator

"*Asian Art Therapists* is an important book that all therapists should read. It raises thought-provoking questions that make therapists from all cultures consider how they may be behaving insensitively to colleagues and clients alike."

Annmarie Grossman, MA, LPC,
PACT program director in NJ, USA

Asian Art Therapists

This book explores Asian art therapist experiences in a predominantly White professional field, challenging readers with visceral, racial, and personalized stories that may push them far beyond their comfort zone.

Drawing from the expertise and practices of Asian art therapists from around the world, this unique text navigates how minority status can affect training and clinical practice in relation to clients, co-workers, and peers. It describes how Asian pioneers have broken therapeutic and racial rules to accommodate patient needs and improve clinical skills and illustrates how the reader can examine and disseminate their own biases. Authors share how they make their own path—by becoming aware of the connection between their lives and circumstances—and how they liberate themselves and those who seek their services.

This informative resource for art therapy students and professionals offers non-Asian readers a glimpse at personal and clinical experiences in a White-dominated profession while detailing how Asian art therapists can lead race-based discussions with empathy to become more competent therapists and educators in an increasingly diversifying world.

Megu Kitazawa, MA, ATR-BC, LCAT, is a NY State Licensed Creative Arts Therapist and Board-Certified Art Therapist currently living in Berlin, Germany, and conducting individual art therapy consultations and workshops for the Japanese and English-speaking expats.

Asian Art Therapists
Navigating Art, Diversity, and Culture

Edited by Megu Kitazawa

Routledge
Taylor & Francis Group

NEW YORK AND LONDON

First published 2021
by Routledge
52 Vanderbilt Avenue, New York, NY 10017

and by Routledge
2 Park Square, Milton Park, Abingdon, Oxon, OX14 4RN

Routledge is an imprint of the Taylor & Francis Group, an informa business

Library of Congress Cataloging-in-Publication Data

Names: Kitazawa, Megu, editor.
Title: Asian art therapists: navigating art, diversity and culture/ edited by Megu Kitazawa.
Description: New York, NY: Routledge, 2021. |
Includes bibliographical references and index.
Identifiers: LCCN 2020026674 (print) |LCCN 2020026675 (ebook) |
ISBN 9780367352660 (hardback) | ISBN 9780367625481 (paperback) |
ISBN 9781003109648 (ebook)
Subjects: LCSH: Art therapy–Cross-cultural studies. | Arts–Therapeutic use–Cross-cultural studies. | Psychotherapists–Attitudes. | Asian Americans–Psychology.
Classification: LCC RC489.A7 A85 2021 (print) | LCC RC489.A7 (ebook) |
DDC 616.89/1656–dc23
LC record available at https://lccn.loc.gov/2020026674
LC ebook record available at https://lccn.loc.gov/2020026675

ISBN: 978-0-367-35266-0 (hbk)
ISBN: 978-0-367-62548-1 (pbk)
ISBN: 978-1-003-10964-8 (ebk)

Typeset in Times NR MT Pro
by KnowledgeWorks Global Ltd.

Contents

List of figures   ix
Acknowledgments   xi
Contributors   xii

Introduction: Unsettling Matter of Race and Ethnicity   1

MEGU KITAZAWA

1 History Matters: Stories about Identity, Culture,
  and Art Therapy   9

JAYASHREE GEORGE

2 The Portrait of a Color-Blind Art Therapist: A Japanese Art
  Therapist Working with Minority Clients in NYC   25

MEGU KITAZAWA

3 Returning to the Sacred Circle, Immigrant
  and Indigenous Allies: A Heuristic Perspective   41

SHEBA SHEIKHAI

4 My Optional Practical Training Experience: My Perspective
  as a Japanese Art Therapy Student   55

HARUKA KAWATA

5 An Art Therapist's Perspective on Cultural Humility in Diverse Setting: A Personal Journey from India to the United States of America   65

SANGEETA PRASAD

6 Between Melting Pots: A Filipino American Art Therapist and the Bean Project   75

MARIA ALINEA-BRAVO

7 Unrealistic Expectations and Harsh Realities: Navigating Career Development as an Asian Art Therapist   83

ASHLEY SEVERSON

8 Find Lost Name: Self-Reflection on the Journey of Being an Art Therapist   93

CHIA-LING KAO

9 Interweaving Art, Therapy, and Cultural Diversity   107

SUNHEE K. KIM

10 Intracultural Practice for Asian Art Therapists: "Are You One of Us, or Are You One of Them?"   121

MIKI GOERDT

11 Possible Use of Art-Based Supervision in Japan   139

REIKO FUJISAWA

Conclusion: A Need for Cognitive Diversity in Multicultural Training   151

MEGU KITAZAWA

Index   155

Figures

1.1 *Shree Ganeshaya Dhimahi.* Acrylic on canvas
by Jayashree George 13
1.2 *Under Ganesha's gaze.* Mixed media by Jayashree George 13
1.3 The detail of *Under Ganesha's Gaze* by Jayashree George 14
2.1 Sumi Ink example by Megu Kitazawa 32
2.2 Sumi Ink example by Megu Kitazawa 32
2.3 Sumi Ink example by Megu Kitazawa 33
2.4 Sumi Ink example by Megu Kitazawa 33
2.5 *Portrait of Megu* by an adult patient in a NYC
psychiatric hospital 34
2.6 *Portrait of Megu* by an adult patient in a NYC
psychiatric hospital 35
2.7 *Portrait of Megu* by an adult patient in a NYC
psychiatric hospital 35
2.8 *Portrait of Megu* by an adult patient in a NYC
psychiatric hospital 36
2.9 *A patient's Geisha image* by Megu Kitazawa drawn from
her memory 37
2.10 *Japan festival* poster in Berlin. Photograph taken by Megu
Kitazawa 38
3.1 *Stage 7: Squaring the Circle* by Sheba Sheikhai 42
3.2 *Chameleon, Stage 11: Fragmentation* by Sheba Sheikhai 44
3.3 *Mni Wiconi*, Stage 3: Labyrinth/Spiral by Sheba Sheikhai 46
3.4 *Duality* by Sheba Sheikhai 47
3.5 *Negotiation*, Stage 6: Dragon Fight by Sheba Sheikhai 49
3.6 *Diversity Continuum* by Sheba Sheikhai 50
3.7 *Self-Portrait*, Stage 5: Target by Sheba Sheikhai 51
3.8 *Knowing* by Sheba Sheikhai 53
4.1 Drawing by Haruka Kawata 58
4.2 Drawing by Haruka Kawata 59
5.1 Drawing by a child in a school 69
5.2 Drawing by a child in a school 70

5.3	Drawing by a child in a school	71
5.4	Drawing by a child in a school	71
5.5	Drawing by a child in a school	72
6.1	Art project by a resident in a nursing home, NYC	79
6.2	Art project by a resident in a nursing home, NYC	80
6.3	Art project by a resident in a nursing home, NYC	80
6.4	Combined works by the participants	81
7.1	Drawing by Ashley Severson	84
7.2	Drawing by Ashley Severson	87
8.1	*Beneath The Anger* by Chia-Ling Kao	99
8.2	*My Daily Art Journals: Drawing Emotions* by Chia-Ling Kao	100
8.3	*Depression and I* by Chia-Ling Kao	101
8.4	*Depression and I* by Chia-Ling Kao	102
8.5	*The Breakthrough Moments* by Chia-Ling Kao	103
8.6	*Those Little Joys And Tears* by Chia-Ling Kao	104
8.7	*The Journey, To Be Continued* by Chia-Ling Kao	105
9.1	Mrs. H.'s expressive writings on the back of her paintings	109
9.2	*Longing for My Homeland.* Acrylic painting in oriental style by a patient	110
9.3	*A Woman Enjoying Spring Breeze.* Acrylic painting by a patient	112
9.4	*He Needs Help.* Acrylic painting by a patient	113
9.5	*Korea*, Acrylic painting by a patient	115
9.6	*No Drink*, Acrylic painting by a patient	116
9.7	*Sky Has No Borders.* Acrylic painting by Sunhee K. Kim	118
9.8	*My New York City.* Acrylic painting by a patient	119
10.1	*Cultural Identity.* Drawing by Miki Goerdt	129
10.2	*Self-portrait.* Drawing by Miki Goerdt	130
10.3	*Drawing of Anxiety in a Container* by a client	132
10.4	*Dot Mandala* by a client	133
11.1	*What Provokes My Anxiety.* Drawing by a supervisee	145
11.2	*Untitled.* Drawing by a supervisee	146
11.3	*Untitled.* Drawing by a supervisee	147

Acknowledgments

I would like to thank the American Art Therapy Association (AATA) conference committee for selecting my focus group, "The Voices of Asian Art Therapists," for its 2018 annual conference. Through this opportunity, Amanda Devine, editor at Routledge, reached out to us and proposed the idea for this book. I would also like to thank Yasmine Awais, my oldest colleague, whose research about cultural diversity, race, and ethnicity in the field of art therapy I deeply respect.

I would also like to thank my German family, Werner, Gerda and Christian Butte for their support in taking care of my children while I was away at art therapy conferences.

Last but not least, I would like to express my highest respect and gratitude to the contributors to this book. You have been courageous in translating your personal experiences into these narratives. Thank you.

Megu Kitazawa, MA, ATR-BC, LCAT

Contributors

Maria Alinea-Bravo, MA, ATR-BC, LCAT, is a licensed creative arts therapist, who is a Filipina American. She lived most of her life in New York and worked in a psychiatric hospital. She has been working in rehabilitation and nursing care center for 20 years.

Reiko Fujisawa, MA, ATR-BC, LCAT, is a Japanese art therapist who worked in NYC for 16 years. Currently, she works at the Hague Convention Division at the Ministry of Foreign Affairs of Japan as a child psychology specialist, a psychotherapist for teenagers and adults at TELL, and a faculty of Japan International Program of Art Therapy in Tokyo.

Miki Goerdt, LCSW, ATR-BC, is a Japanese clinical social worker, an art therapist, and an artist. She has a private practice in Virginia. She also teaches at George Mason University's Master of Social Work program.

Jayashree George, DA, ATR-BC, is an assistant professor in the Art Therapy Counseling Program at Southern Illinois University Edwardsville (SIUE). She is an art therapist and a marriage and family therapist. An anti-oppression stance is a key part of her clinical, artistic, and scholarly work.

Chia-Ling Kao, MA, MPS, ATR-BC, LCAT, is from Taiwan, and currently works at shelters in Brooklyn, New York. With her Social Work and Education backgrounds, she has been developing research regarding art therapy and social justice for the underprivileged and community change.

Haruka Kawata is a Japanese Master's program student in the Art Therapy Counseling program at Southern Illinois University Edwardsville

(SIUE). She has worked as a behavioral health technician, and she is currently an art therapy intern at BJC Hospice in St. Louis.

Sunhee K. Kim, PhD, ATR-BC, LCAT, teaches graduate art therapy students at Seoul Women's University in Korea. Kim completed her Ph.D. in Expressive Therapies at Lesley University in 2010. Currently, she is serving as an editorial board member for the *Arts in Psychotherapy Journal*, as well as for the *Korean Journal of Art Therapy*.

Megu Kitazawa, MA, ATR-BC, LCAT, is a Japanese art therapist who worked in NYC psychiatric hospitals for 17 years and had a private practice. She became a certified psychoanalytic psychotherapist from Object Relations Institute in 2010. Currently, she conducts private art therapy consultations in the Japanese community in Berlin, Germany.

Sangeeta Prasad, MA, ATR-BC, was born in Chennai, India. She is the co-founder of Circle Art Studio in Virginia, and vice president of the Prasad Family Foundation. She has published two books, *Creative Expressions: Say it with Art* and *Using Art Therapy with Diverse Populations Crossing Cultures and Abilities.*

Ashley Severson, MA, ATR-P, is a Filipina American and works at Maui Youth and Family Services with substance abused teens on the island of Maui, Hawaii. She graduated from the Art Therapy program at The George Washington University in 2019 and moved to Hawaii in hopes of providing art therapy services to people on the island.

Sheba Sheikhai, MA, LGPAT, LGPC, is a Gurkha Indian art therapist. She works as an art therapist at a women's day shelter, and as an artist-in-residence at a behavioral health center in Baltimore, MD, serving the Urban Native American community.

Introduction

Unsettling Matter of Race and Ethnicity

Megu Kitazawa

This book is our first attempt to gather narratives from Asian art therapists. It is a collection of visceral, racial, and personalized experiences that may be uncomfortable for some to read, as discussions of race and ethnicity can be unsettling. Savneet Talwar once said, "Such conversations are difficult and uncomfortable. Although safe spaces are important, I suggest that experiences of discomfort can be transformative" (2015, p. 101). When I started working on this book, I reached out to AATA's Open Forum for contributors to this book to bring a positive transformation to our field. One Asian art therapist, who turned down the offer to be a part of this project, warned me to be careful because of the racial focus of this book. For too long in my career as an art therapist have I been "careful" to continue avoiding the discussion around race and ethnicity. So I decided to move forward with this book because it is time to share "the power of our personal narratives in defining our experiences" (Talwar, 2015, p. 102) with our colleagues.

For a long time, I considered myself to be an American who was born in Japan. I lived in a small city called Hachioji in the Greater Tokyo metropolitan area, where it was safe for children to go to schools and playgrounds and to run errands alone. In the 1980s, J-pop was thriving, manga and anime blossomed, and Hollywood movies were made increasingly available in movie theaters and on VCR cassettes. Traditional practices such as tea ceremonies, Ikebana (Japanese flower arrangement), and wearing Kimonos were far and few between, saved only for special occasions.

I left Japan before I was exposed to issues like gender inequality in workplaces, sexual harassment and abuse of power toward women, and issues with illegal immigrants in Japan. My family structure was unconventional; my mother was a single parent raising two daughters. As such, I was unaware of the harsh reality of single parenting in Japan, especially for women.

In 1989, I moved to the United States to live with my father and attended high school in Pennsylvania. People welcomed me and often asked, "Where are you from?" I received positive support from school personnel and fellow students, which helped with a smooth adjustment and transition into the English-speaking world. There were few other non-White students in the entire cohort of over 200: two African-Americans, a Brazilian exchange student, and a South Korean. I learned how to be American from the community by trying to speak up, to be myself, and to not be timid in developing "a sense of personal identity, self-actualization, locus of control, and post-conventionalism" (Calisch, 2003, p. 13). This process of Americanization led me to abandon my cultural heritage. I eventually stopped reading, speaking, and writing in Japanese and avoided contact with Japanese people.

After 2 years in Pennsylvania, I moved to New York City (NYC) and went to high school in Chinatown. The student body consisted of 20 percent Blacks and Hispanics and 80 percent Chinese and other Asians. I was, yet again, the only Japanese student in the entire school. I behaved as if I were a true-bred American—as American as my friends who were actually born and raised in the United States. Most of my friends initially thought I was Chinese because they had never met a Japanese attending public school in the middle of Chinatown before. I did not fit into their pre-conceptualized knowledge about Japanese teenagers, which was that they attended private schools in either Scarsdale or Westchester, NY.

I started studying art therapy in 1998 and experienced a drastic change in my surroundings, going from a mainly Chinese, Black, and Hispanic environment to having frequent interactions with White female students and professors. Again, my ethnicity was never an issue because of their openness to include me. One weekend, I took a "multicultural" course that stirred up mixed feelings. I went into it excited, thinking that it was about race and ethnicity and that it would be a platform on which I could share and address how differently I looked and felt. But I ended up learning mostly about people with disabilities, the deaf culture, and a White art therapist from Europe. The instructor was even more surprised when I did not work on a making of Geisha, when we did art experiential learning about one's heritage. Needless to say, I was disappointed with the course. This experience also woke me up to the alternate reality that I had created—one in which I was a White American—and made me realize that I was not as Americanized as I thought; people still viewed me as a Geisha doll or someone who liked wearing Kimonos. Despite this realization, I wasn't ready to deal with the truth. My defense mechanism kicked in and I retreated into my comfort zone: my state of denial, intentionally oblivious to the color of my skin, hair, and facial complexion. Thus far, I had gained no "knowledge," "awareness," nor "skills" (Acton, 2001, p. 111) needed to be a competent multicultural art therapist.

In 2007, I was studying at a psychoanalytic institute. My White male supervisor approached me and recommended a chapter written by Narumi Taniguchi (2005) from a book called *Voices of Color: First-Person*

Accounts of Ethnic Minority Therapists. He thought it would be "interesting" for me to read something written by a Japanese family therapist. In doing so, my supervisor made no mention of ethnicity, race, or my Japanese heritage. Neither did I want to discuss my being a non-White clinician, so that promptly marked the end of our transient conversation about ethnicity and race.

The article survived multiple re-locations and remained in my storage file for another 10 years. I reread the article much later when I was slowly accepting my non-White status and starting to embrace my Japanese heritage. It was titled "From Polarization to Pluralization: The Japanese Sense of Self and Bowen Theory" and it was based on Murray Bowen's family systems theory. In it, Taniguchi described how she helped to create a sense of self for patients with whom she held couples therapy sessions. But Taniguchi spoke little about her personal experiences and feelings about treating White patients and how they reacted to being treated by a Japanese woman. It seemed oddly distant from my own experience. Though we were both Japanese, I was unable to relate.

In the meantime, I found Jayashree George's article by accident. She is an Indian art therapist and an educator of color. In 2005, she wrote "Three Voices on Multiculturalism in the Art Therapy Classroom" in the *Journal of the American Art Therapy Association*, in which she talked about her teaching experiences. The article focused on "first-person narratives that emerged from classroom discussions about privilege, White experience, cultural encounters, and achieving cultural competence" and how her ethnic background, in being different from her students, resulted in "heightening the complexity of the learning situation" (George Greene, & Blackwell, 2005, p. 133). The article showcased her personal narratives and was a very refreshing read in the journal, and one that I could comprehend and empathize with.

I finally finished reading *Voices of Color* in 2016 as I was preparing to write a proposal for a focus group at AATA's annual conference, which was accepted for the 2018 conference in Miami. Called "Voices of Asian Art Therapists," the session was aimed at discussing what it was like to be Asian in the field of art therapy. Though the 45-minute session proved too short to really tackle the issue in depth and raise awareness, we received much heartening support from those with minority backgrounds and statuses in our field, who encouraged us to continue addressing this pressing matter. The motivation of my focus group was similar to that of *Voices of Color*. As explained by its authors, Rastogi and Wieling (2005), "Our literature search revealed that, barring a few exceptions, a strong, first-person voice of therapists of color was missing from the literature," and that the book was meant to "record and disseminate these perspectives by documenting the experiences of therapists of color" (p. 2).

All of the contributors to this book are female as it reflects the demographic in our profession. In this book, we refer to "Asians" as people from China, Japan, South Korea, India, the Philippines, and Southeast Asia. We do not cover all Asian countries in the continental sense of the word nor people who are mixed race and identify as Asians. In addition, it is important to note that many of us have lived in the United States for a long time and consider ourselves as Asian Americans. As such, the focus of this book derives more from an "American" perspective instead of, for instance, a Japanese learning and practicing art therapy in Japan. We also lack the diversity of therapists *Voices of Color* has, which includes Latino therapists, a therapist with Mohawk ancestry, African-American mental health professionals, Muslim therapists, and Hindu family therapists. We also acknowledge the lack of other contentious topics such as political and gender oppression, sexual orientation, gender issues, socio-economic status, disability, and religious and spiritual diversity.

The authors of this book agree and acknowledge that these collective narratives do not apply to all Asian art therapists or the experiences of other Asian mental health professionals. Chapter 1, "History Matters: Stories about Identity, Culture, and Art Therapy," is written by Jayashree George, who unpacks her identities by introducing multiple layers of the history of caste-based discrimination in India and during its 200 years of British rule. Her search for identity had important ramifications not only on her role as an art therapist but also as an educator, teaching graduate-level students who were mostly White Americans. George also opens up the practice of art therapy classes that are mostly held behind closed doors, which prevents us from knowing what really goes on in these sessions.

In Chapter 2, "The Portrait of a Color-Blind Art Therapist: A Japanese Art Therapist Working with Minority Clients in NYC" by Megu Kitazawa, the author describes her art therapy and psychoanalysis training. The textbook instructions she received in her classes did not help her grow because she was a color-blind art therapist. The chapter touches on how she felt frustrated with innocuous misunderstandings, being stereotyped by other professionals, and her struggles with her bicultural identity.

Issues of cultural identity are discussed throughout the book by the authors—both directly and indirectly as in the following chapters. In Chapter 3, "Returning to the Sacred Circle, Immigrant and Indigenous Allies: A Heuristic Perspective" by Sheba Sheikhai, the author talks about her search for her ancestral Northeast Indian and Buddhist roots and her holistic healing approach with the use of a sacred symbol, the mandala.

Haruka Kawata's piece called "My Optional Practical Training Experience: My Perspective as a Japanese Art Therapy Student" in Chapter 4 is based on an interaction the author had with a client who misidentified her as a Chinese when she was an art therapy student. The reflective process she took following the incident led her to start creating art that increased self-awareness and encouraged mutual empathy with the client. From this chapter we might notice that when learning about diversity and multiculturalism, achieving self-awareness is easier said than done. One of the ways to increase self-awareness is introduced by Sangeeta Prasad in Chapter 5 "An Art Therapist's Perspective on Cultural Humility in Diverse Setting: A Personal Journey from India to the United States of America." The author talks about her supervision and work experiences to provide readers with lessons on cultural humility and tips on how to be humble to one's culture as well as others'.

Chapter 6, "Between Melting Pots: A Filipino American Art Therapist and the Bean Project" by Maria Alinea-Bravo, is a delightful, art-based narrative about the author's use of beans. The Bean Project encouraged her participants to bond and helped Maria open up to their cultural backgrounds and be more receptive and humble to their diversity. But having a family doesn't always mean having support and encouragement. In Chapter 7, "Unrealistic Expectations and Harsh Realities: Navigating Career Development as an Asian Art Therapist" by Ashley Severson, the author shares her family history and their disapproval of her career choice as an art therapist. She also talks about her peers' perception of her as someone who was not White but deemed "White enough" because of her upbringing. Is it easier to become a recognized art therapist when one is born as a White American?

This question brings us to Chapter 8, a heartbreaking story written by Chia-Ling Kao. In "Find Lost Name: Self-Reflection on the Journey of Being an Art Therapist," the Taiwanese art therapist describes how she used narrative art therapy techniques to recover from depression. Her emotional hardships, from struggling to find a job to being a victim of sexual assaults and harassment at work, awe readers and commands empathy. This empathic stance is crucial for learning about racial diversity in art therapy and contributing to a book like this.

Cases of Asian art therapists working with minority clients, including those with an Asian background, are more common than one thinks. In Chapter 9, "Interweaving Art, Therapy, and Cultural Diversity," by Sunhee Kim, the author describes her intercultural practice as a therapist in which her cultural background is different from her clients'. She discusses how she adopted Carl Rogers' teachings of empathic listening and unconditional positive regard concept to help her speak openly about the differences between her and her clients and how that approach not only transformed them but also herself.

Author Miki Goerdt considers the flip side of the coin, the so-called intracultural practice, in Chapter 10, "Intracultural Practice for Asian Art Therapists: "Are You One of Us, or Are You One of Them?"." She raises the question, "Are you one of us, or are you one of them?" and shares her clinical expertise of intra-cultural practice and the incidences of same-race misunderstandings. She applauds the bicultural competencies of Asian art therapists equipped with Western art therapy training in treating clients of the same race.

The globalization of art therapy is still a concept that is hard to grasp. With limited training programs and resources, art therapists trained in the United States will continue to face challenges when practicing in their home countries. Final Chapter 11 describes such an ordeal by Reiko Fujisawa and is titled "Possible Use of Art-Based Supervision in Japan." Reiko describes her return to Japan and surprised at discovering how unacknowledged and underutilized art-based supervision there remains. This informative piece also briefly introduces us to Japan's unsatisfactory mental health system. Today, Reiko continues to advocate the importance of a life-long learning process and art-based supervision for non-art therapy clinicians.

It's been 18 years since Abby Calisch wrote, "The minority membership within the profession of art therapy is quite underrepresented," and, "Art therapists from minority cultures are so few that they could not address the service needs of the populations they represent, even if their practices were solely restricted to their own cultures" (2003, p. 12). It's also been 6 years since Yasmine Awais stated, "The current situation of predominately White students being educated by predominantly White faculty may be problematic in the treatment of non-White populations" (Awais & Yali, 2015, p. 115). That causes some discordance with not only the treatment of non-Whites but also the education of non-White art therapists. I hope to see progress in our field in 2021. Let's forget what we have learned about focusing on "individuals and their presenting problems and symptoms," (Lee, 2005, p. 91), and the belief that a "therapeutic encounter is immune to racism" (p. 96). Our future lies in learning to use our voices to discuss racial and ethnic issues in our classroom and clinical settings, and creating a safe place for art making. I am neither a scientific nor an academic researcher. Still, I hope for this book to become a new resource for students and professionals and for it to offer a glimpse of our personal and clinical experiences as Asian art therapists.

References

Acton, D. (2001). The "color blind" therapist. *Art Therapy: Journal of the American Art Therapy Association, 18*(2), 109–112. http://dx.doi.org/10.1080/07421656.20 01.10129749

Awais, Y., & Yali, A. M. (2015). Efforts in increasing racial and ethnic diversity in the field of art therapy. *Art Therapy: Journal of the American Art Therapy Association, 32*(3), 112–119. https://doi.org/10.1080/07421656.2015.1060842

Calisch, A. (2003). Multicultural training in art therapy: Past, present, and future. *Art Therapy: Journal of the American Art Therapy Association, 20*(1), 11–15. http://dx.doi.org/10.1080/07421656.2003.10129632

George, J., Greene, B. G., & Blackwell, M. (2005). Three voices on multiculturalism in the art therapy classroom. *Art Therapy: Journal of the American Art Therapy Association, 22*(3), 132–138. https://doi.org/10.1080/07421656.2005.10129492

Lee, L. J. (2005). Taking off the mask: Breaking the silence–the art of naming racism in the therapy room. In M. Rastogi, & E. Wieling (Eds.), *Voices of color: First-person accounts of ethnic minority therapists* (pp. 91–115). Sage Publications.

Rastogi, M., & Wieling, E. (2005). Introduction. In M. Rastogi, & E. Wieling (Eds.), *Voices of color: First-person accounts of ethnic minority therapists* (pp. 1–9). Sage Publications.

Talwar, S. (2015). Culture, diversity, and identity: From margins to center. *Art Therapy: Journal of the American Art Therapy Association, 32*(3), 100–103. https://doi.org/10.1080/07421656.2015.1060563

Taniguchi, N. (2005). From polarization to pluralization: The Japanese sense of self and Bowen theory. In M. Rastogi, & E. Wieling (Eds.), *Voices of color: First-person accounts of ethnic minority therapists* (pp. 265–276). Sage Publications.

1 History Matters

Stories about Identity, Culture, and Art Therapy

Jayashree George

Psychology exhorts us to "Know Thyself." Underlying notions of self-knowledge, the necessity of self-reflection undergirds theoretical concepts such as transference, countertransference, and projective identification whose relevance is found beyond their origins in psychoanalysis. Self-knowledge is also a cornerstone of ethical practice. It is in the spirit of such a reflective practice that I present stories about identity, culture, and art therapy as a cis-gender, South Asian, female family art therapist-educator.

"Is my art Indian?" I asked, during my first semester in the art therapy program in the United States. I had asked the rhetorical question out loud when I was in the company of my friend, who was White, as I mused about my art products. It sounded nonsensical. My question/concern was embedded in the context of all that I had just experienced in my studies over the past 5 years in Fine Arts in India. My friend responded, "Look at yourself in the mirror." It was awfully glib—"If you are from _____ (India), your art must be _____ (Indian) as well." There was a context to my question, and it seemed misplaced in the context of the United States. It is this context that underlies my identity as it was shaped in India before it encountered further re-shaping in the United States. The rest of this chapter is an unpacking of these contexts.

When I was 15, I had my debut performance in Bharatanatyam, a classical Indian dance, at the House of Soviet Culture in Mumbai, India. About three quarters of the way through the performance, I remember being on stage, seated alongside the two chief guests for the event. In their speeches, I heard them both talk about "India's hoary culture," and I wondered, "What does 'hoary' mean?" I made a mental note to look it up after the performance. But even more, I wondered, "I know I am a dancer and I am Indian, I have learned Indian dance. That's a part of our culture. But, what does culture really mean? They have said the word 'culture' so many times! What IS Indian culture?" At 15, I did not realize how much I had been swimming in culture, that only getting out of it could help me articulate to myself what culture in all its layered meanings could represent for me. The rest of this chapter will elucidate these layers. By the way, I looked up the word "hoary"—in short, it means "ancient," "venerable," and it is a reference to grayish-white or silvery hair, referring to a person's advancing years. I decided that "ancient" and "venerable" were apt descriptions.

Barely 3 years later, at 18, I was standing in line, struggling to get admission into college. I had good grades. There was no reason to not get in, or so I thought. I had moved from one Southern State in India to another. Suddenly, my being Brahmin, one of the upper-caste groups in India where casteism is practiced with fervor even today, was a problem. India had made a decision to have quotas for lower-caste individuals, who had historically been oppressed, in order to level the playing field for all. This point was lost on me. All I knew at my young age was that I did not get accepted and I felt elbowed out of the way by the quota system.

The vigor of caste-based discrimination in India, despite laws prohibiting it, and the fervor of Brahmins (upper-caste individuals) feeling victimized by the laws, is only matched by White supremacy in the United States. In Mumbai, in Western India, it was different than in Chennai, in Southern India. I had felt relatively removed from caste-based consciousness in Mumbai, while in Chennai, I was thrust into the thick of it. I felt a lot of self-pity and righteous indignation. In 2019, news about the college admissions scandal broke in the United States where ultra-rich parents had invented all sorts of ways to get their children into high-profile schools because they felt that affirmative action had precluded access for their children (Taylor, 2019). There appeared to be no difference between my lack of caste consciousness so many years ago and the current elitism of the ultra-rich: one was caste-based supremacy or being "too Brahmin," the other was classist, or being "too rich," and where classism exists alongside racism. I had come into contact with the caste aspect of my identity and the unearned privileges I had inherited even as I was blind to these inheritances. Caste is part and parcel of Hindu culture even as laws forbid it. In fact, I remember going to a meeting at the Theosophical Society, a venerated place in Chennai that had been avant-garde in its time for its support of Indian independence from British rule. The leaders discussed how Brahmins were now being victimized, a dominant narrative that marks Indian politics today. This is not unlike the contemporary narrative in the United States of "the-war-on-Christmas" and saving "Real-America" for "real-Americans" which is code for preserving White supremacy, including preservation of Christianity, which goes against the core of "e pluribus unum" (out of many, one), the motto of the United States.

History matters. It informs the things we do in ways that feel "normal," or "natural," and makes us perform in automaticity, more than one would like to admit. For example, the story of my opportunity to learn dance could be told in two ways. In the first narrative, I could say, "I did not realize that my opportunity to learn dance was a part of reformation in post-colonial India where the ravages of colonialism had, on the one hand, killed the feudal patronage of the arts, especially dance and the performing arts, which were caste-specific. On the other hand, the British rule did attempt to put an end to casteism, but the British lived their class-saturated lives, equivocating about equality." This might be seen as a colonial retelling. Another way to tell the same story using Sreebitha's (2014) analysis is thus: "I did not realize that my opportunity to learn dance came as a result of the appropriation of *sadir*, a devadasi (lower caste) dance form, that was appropriated by upper-caste women to be taught to upper-caste women while they 'destroyed the very art forms they have borrowed from' (Sreebitha, 2014, p. 7)." Even as the British were trying to end casteism, reformation was being dictated by oppressor to the oppressed. And, it is also true that there was caste oppression within the Indians, a practice that dated back centuries. The second narrative problematizes what one might have taken for granted in the aforementioned colonial retelling. I was learning that culture is, in part, tied to place, its history, and the ways people sorted themselves by creating socially dominant methods for the sorting. Thereby, the products of culture are practiced in ways that may or may not be obvious in terms of their historical roots. The irony of my learning dance was that my first teacher was a Muslim woman, who was married to a Sindhi, and who learned a Hindu dance form that was appropriated from *sadir*, by an upper-caste woman, Rukmini Devi Arundale, who was married to a White, British man.

To some extent I was able to answer the questions I had for myself about Indian culture by studying Indian art history as a part of my education in Fine Arts in undergraduate and graduate studies. I finally began to understand the intricate connections between literature, music, dance, and sculpture in Hindu South India. It took leaving India for me to encounter Indian culture and historical heritage in ways I couldn't quite fathom while I was immersed in the ocean that is Indian culture. Even as I write this, I wonder, which Indian culture? Hindu culture? Brahmanical culture? Middle-class culture in South India? Perhaps it would be more appropriate to say, "my Indian culture" which is Brahmin, middle-class, Southern, urban, mixed a little bit with Catholic traditions from being in Jesuit institutions for the entirety of my education. And this means that I have no authority to speak for any other Indian on the basis of caste, religion, community, geographical location, or indigenous heritage, for India is an extremely diverse people.

Five years after art school in Southern India, I found myself in the United States, studying art therapy. In art school in India, while we were studying modern Indian art in the late eighties, we were told to inquire about what was Indian art. Traditional Indian art had fallen into disuse during British rule (including the rise of the East India company) that lasted from the mid-eighteenth century until 1947. The British period was governed by a legacy of watered-down neo-classical art that had primacy over traditional Indian art that was seen as "primitive," "vulgar," or otherwise savage. Revival of Indian art from the 1920s focused on the question of defining Indian art. Was it traditional, as in pre-British? Was aping the West not Indian? Did the themes have to be Indian? Was art that was classical not as important as art that dealt with the urgency of social issues that needed representation? Even more fundamental was the question, "What constitutes our voice as Indians, especially after being colonized for over 200 years?"

During British times, traditional Indian art was seen as inferior by the British. In fact, just recently, an exhibition of "Company Paintings" at the Wallace Collection in London, curated by William Dalrymple, was reviewed by Verma (2020):

> Paintings commissioned by patrons of the East India Company during the late 18th and early 19th Centuries ... focuses on artists who were previously neglected .... It seems remarkable that work of such brilliance has been neglected—but their labelling means they've been caught in limbo, as Dalrymple tells BBC Culture, "They're toxic to both India and Britain—to India they're not Indian enough, they reek of colonialism, and for Britain there's an embarrassment around Empire. After the collapse of Empire, the British put this thing in a trunk in the attic and forgot about it."

Therefore, when I shared my concern during my first semester in the graduate art therapy program in the United States, "Is my art Indian?" it referred to all this history and being out of context, it sounded like nonsense! In the early years, I was cast as decidedly "Indian" in America. I was not my localized identity but subsumed under *all-of-India*. I realized later that I was trying to convey to my friend that I had been steeped in an identity struggle in India on account of my identity as an artist and that the struggle was about post-colonial identity. I hadn't even begun to think about my identity as an Indian in the United States. I was nowhere close to my re-definition as "Indian-American" or "South-Asian-American." Nor had I really begun to unpack my Brahmin identity and its ramifications.

To this day, when I paint, I am self-conscious about my artistic style and technique: how much of it harks back to tradition, of which I was never really a part, except by osmosis, and how much of it is Western, on account of my education? And, it hits hard when I take my work to a gallery and hear a comment like, "It's too ethnic. It won't sell." I also hear comments from fellow Indians who say, "That's cute," when my art is decidedly Indian. In this identity it is hard to win—either I am not Western enough, therefore ethnic, or too Indian even for Indians. Examples of this are two pieces of artwork, Figures 1.1 to 1.3. And then,

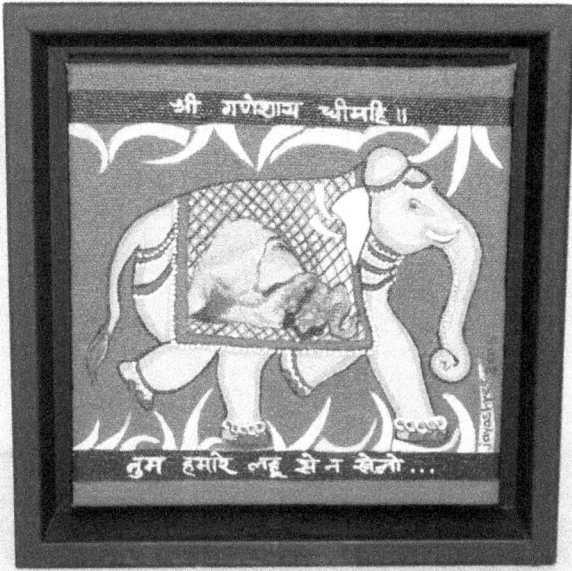

Figure 1.1 Shree Ganeshaya Dhimahi. Acrylic on canvas by Jayashree George.

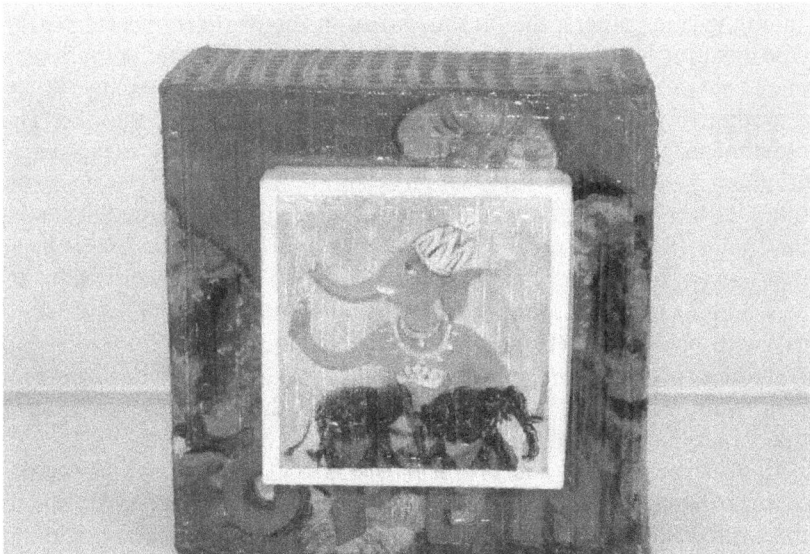

Figure 1.2 Under Ganesha's gaze. Mixed media by Jayashree George.

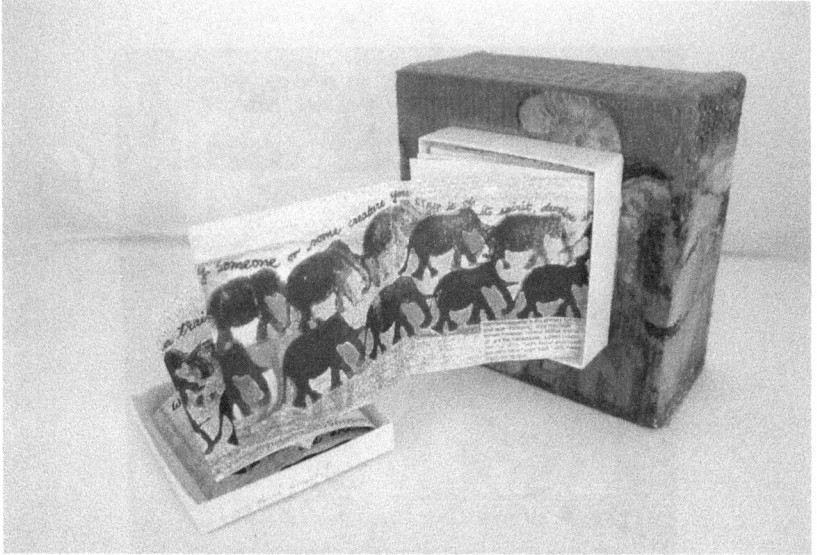

Figure 1.3 The detail of *Under Ganesha's Gaze* by Jayashree George.

I am faced with how much of me is Indian, in terms of ethnicity and how much of me is American as I negotiate my hyphenated existence as Indian American. All three paintings deal with activism to agitate against the poaching of elephants in Asia and Africa.

In considering identity, I found that there are two meanings of it, among various others, that are prevalent in the world of mental health. One meaning has to do with a generic one that may have more to do with one's role or experience of a state, for example, "I am a parent," "I am a mother of a child with autism," "I am depressed," and the like. The other meaning has to do with societally conferred identities, such as race/ethnicity, gender, nationality, sexual orientation, class, etc. It is the latter that I wish to describe. Some authors (Rowe et al., 1994; Sue & Sue, 2008) have suggested that there is a trajectory of minority identity development that moves from unitary identification with one's racial group and ends with a bi- or multi-cultural identity where the individual maintains identity with one's racial/ethnic group and also enjoys an easy relationship with the dominant racial/ethnic group. The key appears to be movement from conflict to harmony and this highlights the acculturation process that values harmony over conflict.

In my experience, I had my identity consolidated before I left India, even as I struggled with the constituent elements of it. When I came to the United States, I found no need to acculturate in the method laid out by the racial and cultural identity development (R/CID) models. I neither flocked to solely South-Asian saturated groups, even as these were available to me quite readily, nor did I disavow South-Asian groups. I did not experience the yearning of wanting to fit in. I was never quite enamored of the United States and moved only because of familial pressure. The American dream was alive for my siblings but seemed nonsensical to me. When I finally decided to stay, it was for pragmatic reasons. I found that my exploration of the differences and similarities in the power structures of Indian and US societies helped me articulate to myself the values by which I would live. Perhaps my facility with language cushioned my acculturation process; however, I am not convinced that a harmonious co-existence with the dominant culture is necessary. What I think might be more valuable is to have critical thinking such that there is greater bandwidth among dominant and non-dominant groups to be able to deal with conflict and difference. Conflict is not necessarily synonymous with disharmony. Harmony that fords conflict is hard won and might actually create stronger bonds as a result of being able to withstand truth telling.

George et al. (2005) write that it is much easier to identify ourselves as victims rather than as oppressors. It is in such examination that we may consider racial and ethnic identity models. In particular, Shin (2015) critiques the R/CID models. While noting their significant contribution and early intent to destabilize universal models of identity, he also notes that these models have fallen into the same canon of universalizing all racial and ethnic identities into one trajectory toward "healthy integration, which includes the acceptance of one's racial/ethnic background as well as a respect for the cultural norms of other groups" (Shin, 2015, pp. 12–13). The hint of assimilationist ideas in the form of "Let's all get along together" seems to hover in the framework. Missing are the jagged trajectories of development in the contexts of Native American genocide, slavery, or the various immigrant contexts, which, Shin says, "leads to implicit pathologizing of the diverse range of life trajectories experienced by individuals" (p. 16) and delegitimizes their justifiable anger. Shin takes pains to clarify the usefulness of the models while also critiquing them and offers an example of one such misuse by a fellow professor during a discussion about a student, noting his place in his ethnic identity development.

Sue and Sue (2008) cite critiques of White racial identity development models, which similarly flow from a state of naivete toward a state of "autonomy" (Helms, 1995) or "integration" (Rowe et al., 1994; Sue & Sue, 2008). Noting the languaging in the end states of each model, we hear familiar refrains of "comfort," "recognition," and a "getting-along-togetherness" that hint toward assimilation (subtext: minorities are digestible) and which value individualism. Here are some examples of the end states of White racial identity development:

> Informed positive socioracial group commitment, use of internal standards for self-definition, capacity to relinquish the privileges of racism ... (as cited in Sue & Sue, 2008, p. 251).

Integrative types "have integrated their sense of whiteness with a regard for racial/ethnic minorities ... [and] integrate rational analysis, on the one hand, and moral principles, on the other, as they related to a variety of racial/ethnic issues" (Rowe et al., 1994, p. 141) (as cited in Sue & Sue, 2008, p. 253).

Sue and Sue's (2008) model includes being aware of sociopolitical influences regarding racism and taking on an anti-oppressive stance, however, when they write, "The person values multiculturalism, is comfortable around members of culturally different groups" (p. 253), even with the caveat that the person will be anti-oppressive, I worry about the very same assimilationist tendencies. When we are not taught to ford conflict, to stay with discomfort when we are trying to be allies, to conduct agent-to-agent conversations, justice will be a casualty. We can fall prey to guilt and dissonance. When we are unable to acknowledge historical facts or able to converse across borders, our very values of democracy, of having the skills to hold opposite ideas, of managing conflict effectively, become threatened. Such a value system is still burgeoning in the mainstream of psychology and counseling and not fully present in the field of art therapy.

My journey in the United States has been a journey unpacking my various identities. In the early years, I had been in an internal, preoccupied state, ruminating on all that had passed. As I looked up, I noticed the different ways in which I was being seen, my image as reflected back to me by others, especially White individuals. At first, when I was in my twenties, it was a focus on my language acquisition:

"You speak English so well."
My response at the time was, "After 200 years of British rule, I had better speak English well." However, in that response, I was leaving out millions of Indians who had resisted the onslaught of English, and had clung to the vernacular, as I had not. I had lost any foothold onto my mother tongue, Tamil-it was a loss.
"Why do you wear a red dot? What does it mean?"
At first, I explained that the red dot was called a bindi and that it was a symbol of womanhood in India, that the circular shape was about wholeness. But, I also explained that it was a signifier that sorted women as available (with the bindi) or widowed when the bindi was not placed on the forehead, which is also a form of social ranking. This caused me to think about my bindi. Finally, I said, "it has become a vanity mark."

Then, it was about exoticization, which took a few forms: "I love India!" "I love Indian food." "I have an Indian friend." The words were often accompanied with adoring looks designed to make me feel special. These positive stereotypes existed alongside teens screaming out their car windows, "Go back where you came from!" It was also during the 1990s, the time of the "dot-busters," an anti-Indian group from New Jersey.

When I first arrived in the art therapy program from India, I presented myself in all my authenticity. I wore Indian clothes and Western clothes, just as I did in India. I wore a bindi, I cooked and ate Indian food, and shared my stories with my peers. At the end of the first semester when I had to start my internship, I began to consider how I might be seen by the children with whom I would work. Would the bindi be a distraction? Would *I* become the topic of conversation instead of keeping the focus on the job to be done? And yet, by virtue of this train of thought, I couldn't present myself in all my authenticity. I decided to go bindi-less so that I could be more available, or so I thought. Over the years, having worked with children, my guess is that had I kept the bindi on, yes, it would have been a distraction, but it may have worn off after some time. Children often tackle the truth more directly and deal with it, while most adults tend to bob and weave. I was not sure that the supporting atmosphere, supervision, peer group, and the larger culture would have the endurance to deal with the differences in order to ride through initial distractions. Perhaps this was truer. I had decided to keep the status-quo comfortable and it went along with "professional etiquette," which excluded Indian clothes as they were considered "costumes" rather than "professional outfits" or clothes "du jour."

In terms of exoticism, it can have deleterious effects for clients when such a stereotype is practiced by supervisors. For example, when I was a new graduate, I got a job working with the elderly in nursing homes. My art therapy services were referred to a woman who was Jewish and who had recently become a resident in a nursing home. She was ambulatory and seemed quite skittish about having to work with me. She said to the nurse who had accompanied me to the first session in order to introduce me and set up the working arrangement, "I don't need therapy." However, the nurse, who seemed to have a relationship with the client that made me defer to her judgment, convinced the client that art therapy would be most appropriate. After a couple of visits that resulted in the client shutting herself in her room refusing to meet with me, I took it up with the treatment team and stated that this client was simply not interested in my services and I wondered if it might have to do with my being Indian. The treatment team supervisor/manager pronounced, "But how could someone not want to work with you? You are a sweet Indian woman." I have to confess that I had no idea at the time, being 26 years old and still new to the United States, how to counter this. I had had no class in multicultural issues. I had no way of articulating for myself my identity such that I could help someone else understand. All I knew in the moment was that while I felt flattered, I did not feel helped or heard or respected. Further, I knew that the client was not feeling heard or respected either. And I felt powerless to do anything because my repeated protests over the next several weeks went unheard. This, until I had the bright idea to involve the family who quickly put an end to the "services" and also validated my hunches about what was happening with their mother, that she did not like foreigners.

Then, during my thirties and forties it was about my gender and ethnic identities, usually observed by White males: "You are sure to get a job because you are Indian and you are a woman. I am just stating a fact." This was in reference to affirmative action that barred discrimination against women and minorities. Being in the mid-West in my thirties, I had turned a blind eye to any discriminatory behaviors such as being followed at a Macy's, having a White storekeeper speak slowly because she assumed that I didn't know English, and having White students say, "You don't need sunscreen because you have melanin."

These experiences came to a head for me in the classroom where I now taught future art therapists. This is where I felt the real reckoning took place and continues to do so. I was asked to teach "Multicultural Issues," a required course in the graduate art therapy curriculum. In the beginning, I had a great deal of anxiety about this course because I felt extremely self-conscious about my immigrant status. I was not a citizen and I felt ill-equipped to counter the waves of supremacist views that would be expressed in class by White students. My internal talk went something like this, "Who am I, a foreigner, to tell American citizens about their own history and about the social dominance in their own country?" Clearly, even after years of staying here, I felt like an outsider because of my lack of privilege on account of nationality—I was not yet a US citizen. It was also a rank conferred to me by this society's ordering of those who have privilege (agents) and those who don't (targets) (Nieto et al., 2010). It made me pay attention to my further education in pedagogy dealing with issues of diversity so that I could build my confidence and capacity as an educator. For example, I was never quite sure my answers were satisfactory when students in my class said the following:

"Don't make me apologize for my Whiteness."

"I'm just a poor farm girl from ____ (rural Mid-west). I did not grow up around Blacks. I will return there and will never run into a Black person. So, why should I have to take this course in Multicultural Issues?"

"I used to be aware of differences and then, one day, I felt so guilty, because I couldn't do anything to change what had happened in this country. So, I just went back. And now you are telling me to feel guilty *again*."

"I am so sick and tired of reading this book (Multicultural textbook) and all the chapters where people are complaining of how bad their situation is and what Whites have done to them. I'm going to burn this book after this class is over."

The common denominator was about members of agent groups, especially along the rank of race/ethnicity, complaining about having to take ownership around the privilege of White supremacy. This is a widespread problem. I began to think about other types of supremacy, such as caste-based supremacy in India. I began to think about how I have to keep dismantling Brahmin supremacy in myself.

How do I keep waking up from my stupor of Brahmin-ness? An acquaintance of mine recounted stories of Brahmin discrimination of lower-caste individuals. This triggered in me a memory of a television program I had watched in India that suddenly clicked within me a consciousness of my own supremacy. The image that stayed within me from that program was of high-caste Kerala Brahmins called Namboothiris. The story went that when a Namboothiri showed up somewhere, persons who were lower caste lowered their gaze, quickly lowered their upper garment, and walked backwards as they swept away their footprints. To me this was the ultimate erasure of a people: to sweep one's identity away such that they no longer laid claim to even their footprints. For me, this one image is enough to keep me going in terms of dismantling Brahmin consciousness. I don't need any more evidence. Fanaticism and fundamentalism of all sorts continue to plague many countries around the world.

I began to talk to my students about the process of waking up. I started to develop curiosity about how that waking-up process happens. Suddenly, I was no longer feeling dread as I walked into the classroom and faced supremacist comments. I could see how it was governed by blindness and I could move toward it with curiosity, even as I did not support such views. I would ask students who were a little further along in their process of waking up to talk to the ones who had not woken up as yet. I began to tell my own story. I was no longer feeling like a foreigner. I was no longer succumbing to divisions that society sets up to pit one set of peoples against another. I began to understand that agents (people with privilege) need to talk to other agents along similar axes of power: race/ethnicity, age, abilities, nationality, class, sexual orientation, gender, religion, indigenous heritage, geographical location, etc. I could use my experience of agency within my context as an Indian who was Brahmin and address White agency/White supremacy in the United States.

Some of my students would tell me, "I am White, but I don't practice racism. I don't discriminate against people of color. So, why do I have to have my face rubbed in this all the time?" One student said it best, "Oh, I finally get it!! You are asking me to not take it personally. That's what I had been doing all the time—even though you told me not to. I am seeing it from a societal view. I am getting it! It's not about me. It's about one group of people and another group and what happened between them." Her revelation was an important step forward in her process.

My attention also turned toward individuals of color in the United States. How do we do the work of empowerment and become strategic about which battles to fight? People have varying reactions to the labels that societal rank places on us. It is really not up to us whether we "like" our rank as agents or targets or not. It is an inheritance we are bequeathed, whether we want it or not. Sometimes the inheritance is by virtue of our births. Sometimes it is acquired (e.g., acquired disability) and sometimes it has to do with societal structuring, such as class or age where one can move in and out of any class stratum due to changing circumstances, or age in and out of privilege based on societal structure. When we encounter agent identities within ourselves, it is hard to identify with being an agent, as the demand for making interventions is greater and it is more guilt-provoking to be a bystander.

One of the pitfalls in teaching classes where multicultural content is the focus is that, often, misunderstandings occur when agents talk to targets along differing axes of power, as in one person talking race and the other talking class, or when Whites and persons-of-color talk about race, targets are often put in the position of educating agents about the oppression they have faced. An example of this can be seen in a PBS town hall meeting moderated by Gwen Ifill (2014) that aired on September 26, 2014, after the Michael Brown shooting in Ferguson, MO. In response to Phillip Agnew of Dream Defenders, a person of color, who said that change needed to happen on a systemic level, a White person said:

> I agree ... middle-class white guys like me haven't lived the African-American life .... I understand this feeling of 'the system isn't fair, it's biased against us,' but then when you start going to this idea that '400 years of repression and this system that is still designed to hurt us and still designed to keep us down,'—that starts feeling to me like racism against me just because of the color of my skin. My parents weren't here 400 years ago. My family arrived here way after the civil war ... we're being blamed for things we didn't cause ... (Ifill, 2014)

The conversation went back to Agnew who had to defend his point of view, even as he did not sound defensive. It would have been more fruitful if the moderator had moved the response to Mayor Brian Fletcher, who had said earlier that despite having grown up in White poverty, one cannot know the true plight that African Americans go through unless one is African American. I suggest that it will be a more fruitful conversation in the context of the United States if Whites talk to each other about race, especially if they are willing to speak the truth about the structural inequalities. This would constitute allyship where agents who are further along in the journey of being awake can help other agents who are still in a state of trance (Nieto et al., 2010).

One might wonder why I am writing about Black-White race relations in a chapter on my South-Asian experience. In the same town hall meeting I reference, Teff Poe, a young musician spoke eloquently about the difference between the black experience and the experiences of other immigrants of color. He said:

> We have an issue where black people aren't that far removed from slavery, you know, and I think that other cultures of people are allowed to establish themselves and they're allowed to deal with the issues of their culture, their community and their race appropriately. Yet when it comes to us, we're told that, you know, uh, "get over it," "stop killing each other." (Ifill, 2014)

This voice is important for me to remember as a South-Asian woman, as this is yet another way in which the system divides people of color because it affords some of us the privilege of mobility, while another sector of peoples is denied that privilege. As a result, we are not able to unite as people of color to struggle together to change the rules of the system. Therefore, I suggest that targets become aware of the limits of their abilities to educate or help wake up their agent peers as it is sure to result in feelings of hurt, oppression, disappointment, despair, and burnout. It is a good idea for targets to reach out to people who are in similar target groups for support. The next step is to strategize how much one can do and when to move on in a wakeful state so that we can conserve our energy for things that will actually make a difference in our lives, such as policy decisions that will have long-term consequences (Nieto et al., 2010).

In the clinical realm, the above idea manifests in the form of underlying racism in the clinical encounter. During a diversity workshop that I co-lead, a clinician who identified herself as Irish American said of a black client, a mother who was irate that her son had been referred for therapy by the school, that she was upset about the client's experience of racism. She said to me, "I was thinking to myself, 'Don't talk to me about oppression. I don't want to hear it. You think I was not upset about my people (the Irish) and the racism we encountered? We were also oppressed.'" What was left unsaid was that the black client could never hope to cross over to being White, while that privilege was afforded to the Italians and the Irish where earlier experiences of racism changed as they could enter the White fold. It was yet another strategy of divide and conquer that kept the wheels of White supremacy turning. It is experiences such as these that can subvert the therapeutic alliance, which is a potent factor (empathy has an effect size of .56) leading toward positive therapeutic outcomes (Miller & Chow, 2020).

As art therapists, there is richness in moving back and forth between micro- and macro-levels, from the contexts of our particular histories and familial contexts to larger societal contexts. We encourage clients to do the same as well. The ideas of agency, targetship, and allyship are important concepts for me in the way I practice. For example, violence within the family is something that tends toward secretiveness. This is a space where clients' stories and our own can intersect and the field is rife with the possibility of countertransference or empathy. For instance, when I worked with clients who were survivors of intimate partner violence (IPV), I had to reckon with my own experience of family violence as well as IPV. What helped me in my decision-making? How could I stay present to a story that was different than my experience? In my case, I left a violent relationship successfully. In many cases, the oppressed stay in abusive situations for a variety of reasons. And, sometimes, when couples decide to work on their relationship and commit to non-violence, transformation is possible.

On a societal level, power and control is the common denominator for violence. In this regard, I found common threads when I painted about the plight of elephants that are killed in massive numbers for their tusks. Around 96 elephants are killed every day. For oppression to happen, a person or animal or living entity has to be considered an object or a thing and thereby robbed of their/its animate qualities or life-affirming properties. When objectified thus, the inane to the most severe forms of violence become possible. In the case of the elephants, it is greed for political power, funded by the currency of tusks, that outweighs the impact of poverty. In the case of IPV, societal oppression, as well as violence toward animals and the planet, one needs to hold the perspective of the personal, familial, societal structures, as well as global or transnational perspectives to understand the ecology of the problem in order to find ecological solutions. Raising one's voice to sound the alarm is the first step.

The elephants walk in a line against a sunset and collapse into an accordion folded book. They are as old as civilization. Our histories and our liberation are bound up with each other—human to animal. History matters. Clients' biographies matter. Our sociocultural history matters, as it provides a larger time line within which familial histories nest. My identity quests in India and the United States continue as countries also change and grow as we shuttle back and forth in time between cultural contexts. I continue my internal work, my waking-up process, in an effort to keep the field clear as I become receptive to client stories and my dialectical practice as an educator. I hope to maintain a generative inquiry as more stories get bravely told and re-authored.

References

George, J., Greene, B., & Key, M. (2005). Three voices on multiculturalism from the art therapy classroom. *Art Therapy: Journal of the American Art Therapy Association*, 22(3), 132–138. https://doi.org/10.1080/07421656.2005.10129492

Helms, J. E. (1995). An update of Helm's white and people of color racial identity models. In J. G. Ponterotto, J. M. Casas, L. A. Suzuki, & C. M. Alexander (Eds.), *Handbook of multicultural counseling* (pp. 181–198). Sage Publications.

Ifill, G. (Co-anchor & Managing Editor). (2014, September 26). America after Ferguson (PBS Special). https://www.pbs.org/video/pbs-indies-america-after-ferguson/

Miller, S. D., & Chow, D. (2020). Psychotherapy's fatal flaw and how to fix it. Light up the couch, episode 80. https://courses.clearlyclinical.com/courses/take/psychotherapys-fatal-flaw/audio/10637030-streaming-downloadable-audio-including-apple-podcasts-and-google-play-links

Nieto, L., Boyer, M. F., Goodwin, L., Johnson, G. R., & Smith, L. C. (2010). *Beyond inclusion beyond empowerment: A developmental strategy to liberate everyone.* Cuetzpalin.

Rowe, W., Bennett, S. K., & Atkinson, D. R. (1994, January). White racial identity models: A critique and alternative proposal. *The Counseling Psychologist, 22*(1), 129–146. https://doi.org/10.1177/0011000094221009

Shin, R. Q. (2015). The application of critical consciousness and intersectionality as tools for decolonizing racial/ethnic identity development models in the fields of counseling and psychology. In Goodman, R. D., & Gorski, P. C. (Eds.). *Decolonizing "multicultural" counseling through social justice* (pp. 10–22). Springer. Kindle Edition.

Sreebitha, P. V. (2014, April 6). Sanskritization or appropriation: Caste and gender in "Indian" music and dance. *Savari.* http://www.dalitweb.org/?p=2499

Sue, D. W., & Sue, D. (2008). *Counseling the culturally diverse: Theory and practice* (5th ed.). John Wiley & Sons, Inc.

Taylor, K. (2019, October 22). Parents paid to open college doors. Now they're spending to limit prison time. *The New York Times.* https://www.nytimes.com/2019/10/03/us/college-admissions-scandal-consultants.html

Verma, R. (2020, February 11). Rediscovering India's forgotten masterpieces. http://www.bbc.com/culture/story/20200207-rediscovering-indias-forgotten-masterpieces

2 The Portrait of a Color-Blind Art Therapist

A Japanese Art Therapist Working with Minority Clients in NYC

Megu Kitazawa

Introduction

I immigrated to the United States in 1989 when I was 16 years old to live with my father. He had immigrated there 10 years earlier and was part of the first generation of immigrants who were born in a foreign country and later became US citizens. I fall into what's known as the 1.25-generation. The 1.25-generation refers to individuals who immigrate to a new country between the age of 13 and 17 years old ("Immigrant generation," n.d.). Understandably, these individuals have a harder time adapting to their new countries, as they must do so with a relatively strong sense of attachment to their home country, which, in my case is Japan. Growing up in Japan in the 1980s, social norms and traditional gender roles were strictly observed. Schoolteachers held the highest authority over education and discipline. Having proper manners, greeting elders politely, and not intruding in other people's everyday lives were considered to be good behaviors. Having spent my most formative years in Japan, I very naturally conformed to these societal and cultural standards. It wasn't until I left that I realized my innate actions and mannerisms fit the Japanese stereotype: I am polite, timid, hardworking, respectful, and punctual, I enjoy Manga and Anime, I love buying gifts even for strangers, and I also very instinctively bow to greet others when I'm in Japan (Afshar, 2017). As a 1.25-generation immigrant, my struggles with my identity and sense of cultural belonging hindered my assimilation. My journey through university and the initial experiences as a practicing Asian art therapist didn't help.

Living in NYC, I often had to deal with stereotypical comments. My co-workers, fellow students, and patients also constantly challenged my ethnic identity in the psychiatric hospitals where I worked. Had I been there as a temporary visitor to the United States, people might have thought, "She's a foreigner. We understand if she can't speak well and she looks so Japanese. She'll go back anyway." But that wasn't the case, and it proved difficult for my colleagues and patients, who didn't know how to deal with someone who was neither a first- nor a second-generation immigrant. Hearing an accentless English from someone who displayed un-American

mannerisms and attitude rattled them and I sensed their unease and apprehension whenever we spoke. I dreaded discussions about ethnicity and race
as they made me uncomfortable. Doby-Copeland (2006), a non-White art
therapist who teaches cultural diversity, once stated, "Several students
have withdrawn from my classes citing dissonance and others have had
emotional reactions to the course content" (p. 174). This is something I res-
onated with on two levels—as a minority student who studied art therapy
and yet still lacked the training and knowledge needed to deal with racial
stereotypes, and as a therapist who often interacted with some patients
with lower levels of education and a more provincial worldview.

At home, it was implicit that issues of race and ethnicity were not to
be spoken of. My father's stand was to refrain from commenting on such
issues as long as there was no danger to my life. He led by example, too.
Not once did he complain about the racial mistreatments he received. He
simply said, "The US is the greatest country. It doesn't matter where you
come from or what your skin color is. If you work hard, you can be successful. You need to be an American." When I tried to explain my identity
struggles as a result of my hair and skin color and what I represented, he
replied, "Don't worry about them. Just work hard." I became more and
more withdrawn and in time, I stopped talking to him about my experiences. When asked, I would just respond with, "Everything's fine, Dad."

Racially Challenged Situations

My first job involved working with children and adolescents in an
inpatient psychiatric hospital in NYC. Patients there were mainly
Dominicans, Puerto Ricans, and African Americans. Their age ranged
from 7 years old to 16 years old. I was often asked racially biased and
stereotypical questions such as why my eyes were narrow and my skin
was yellow. Patients would also mimic the Chinese language and imitate
martial arts moves in front of me. Out on the streets, catcalls were the
daily norm, with plenty of, "Yo, China girl," and "Ni hao ma!" coming my way. Despite my urge to retaliate, I often felt too humiliated and
exhausted to do so. The mask I created for myself, the one I wore to feel
like a "regular White American," and my inhibitions further complicated
the situation. In clinical settings, I struggled to deal with racially charged
comments like, What are you doing here?" "Shouldn't you be working
somewhere else like at a take-out food restaurant or a nail salon?" You
can't be my therapist when you can't speak English!" and "Asians are
all the same, they speak and look the same." From my encounters with
them, I grew to expect such provincial comments only from less educated
people. But there were a few encounters that proved otherwise.

On one occasion, I was left stunned when an educated colleague asked
me, "Can you integrate Buddhist or Zen teaching into your groups?" When
I said that I didn't know anything about Buddhism and Zen practices, she

looked as if I was joking. I held back on commenting on her uninformed supposition. In all likelihood, I probably just rolled my eyes and walked away. Just recently, a White friend in the United Kingdom told me about an unjust complaint she faced at work. Her seemingly innocuous anecdote left me taken aback—not by the nature of the complaint but her role in it. This friend, who teaches fashion in the United Kingdom, was shown a photo of an Asian model by a student from South Korea, to which she remarked, "Oh, she looks just like you." The student filed a complaint with my friend's superior, asserting that my friend made a racist comment and was inappropriate. Defending herself, my friend thought she was trying to compliment on how beautiful she was, like the model. If I were the student, I might also not have understood that the remark was not intended to offend and might also have felt mistreated. I'd probably have wondered, "Was she saying that to humiliate me by saying that all Asians looked the same?" Or "Was she saying it because she genuinely thought I looked as beautiful as the model?" My friend, on the other hand, felt disappointed that the student had gone to the supervisor instead of talking to her about it directly. Such occurrences, misunderstandings or otherwise, happen all the time. But yet no one is talking about them in the field of art therapy. Art therapy is a White female-dominated profession (Awais & Yali, 2015). George (2005) found, "one can say that there will be an overwhelmingly large number of female art therapists from the dominant culture treating persons from diverse cultures" (p. 133). In addition, the 2013 American Art Therapy Association membership survey stated 87.8% of art therapists were White, 93.4% were female, with only 2.7% responders identifying themselves as Asian/Pacific Islander (Elkins & Deaver, 2015, p. 61). When I was undergoing psychoanalytic training, the issue of race was never fully and sufficiently explored. Even though nearly all my instructors and fellow trainees were White, they didn't identify themselves by their ethnic backgrounds but by the psychoanalysis techniques they adopted—Freudians, Kleinians, and Winnicottians.

During my time in NYC, I felt very racially insecure and tried to dissociate my Asian qualities from my identity and fit in with society by pretending I was a White American. Because of this identity struggle, I froze and panicked whenever my patients and co-workers talked about the Japanese culture. People often assumed that I ate sushi every day, that I knew a Geisha (Geishas are prostitutes), that I wore kimonos and owned one in my closet, and that I most certainly have watched "The Last Samurai," "Memoirs of Geisha," and "Lost in Translation." Not knowing how to handle these challenging conversations, my instinctive reaction was to blame them for being ignorant about people around them despite living in a city with a melting pot of cultures. I also believed, through my family and schooling, "all people should be treated equally without acknowledgment of race or culture" (Acton, 2001, p. 109). At times, I felt the urge to ask them, "I've learned to treat you equally, regardless of your skin color. Why can't you reciprocate?"

Failed Verbal Interventions

Even when I took a psychoanalytic approach to tackle these uncomfortable situations, most didn't turn out the way I expected to. I was ingrained with a "traditional thinking that results when therapists assume that existing therapy approaches and techniques are appropriate for all people regardless of their race, ethnicity, or culture" (Doby-Copeland, 2006, p. 177). Here are a few interactions I had with my co-workers and patients.

PERSON A: Do you speak Chinese?
ME: Sounds like you know something about the Chinese culture. Tell me more.
A: You live in Chinatown, don't you?
ME: Let's think about where you want to live.
A: Are you from China?
ME: Let's talk about where we come from. Why don't you go first?
A: Why is your skin so yellow?
ME: Why do you think it is?
A: I don't understand. Do you speak English?
ME: Do you feel like I don't understand you?

Unfortunately, these verbal interventions were far from helpful. They created mistrust and apprehension, which frustrated my patients (and sometimes colleagues). They responded with outbursts like, "Why on earth do I need to tell you about Chinese culture?! Do I look Chinese to you?!" "You are twisting my words like the doctors and nurses do!" "Let me tell you where I come from, it's an evil and terrible place!" (My patients often grew up in neglected and abused homes). I knew I had to clean up my mess, but I didn't know how. In all my years of training, I never learned about using "recovery skills for getting out of trouble when making mistakes while counseling culturally diverse clients" (Doby-Copeland, 2006, p. 176).

In the face of these failed interactions, the Asian in me was trying to bury what surfaced. And I had a very Japanese reaction: I blamed myself. More specifically, I blamed myself for not being a White American art therapist, who I felt would be able to handle the situation better and earn more respect from their colleagues. Eventually, patients stopped attending my groups and co-workers became superficially friendly and hesitant to collaborate. I felt uneasy and sometimes even fearful whenever I bumped into them at the hospital. But instead of trying to mend these relationships, I turned my focus to new patients in my groups. I thought it taboo to talk about race and ethnicity. In addition, I never had an Asian supervisor and thought it was inappropriate to discuss such issues with my White supervisors, whom I felt couldn't relate. As Lee (2005) said, "Therapists are placed in a double bind whether they choose to speak up or remain silent about racism" (p. 98). Having never had the training to confront such situations, I believed that "there was no room to engage in these conversations therapeutically" (p. 91).

I'm Not White

I was named after the character "Meg" from *Little Women*, who in the Japanese edition, was known as "Megu." In my attempt to bury my Japanese identity, I dropped the "u" and asked people to call me "Meg," which sounded more American and manageable. I hated when people asked me about Japanese stereotypes or called me "Megu" because it felt like I was being denied a chance at being a White American. My anger stemmed from my efforts to hide my insecurities about being Asian. By doing that, I was subconsciously placing them in the same category to treat them equally, as a "color-blind" art therapist, instead of considering their racial and ethnic backgrounds.

Since it was futile to confide in my father about the issues I was facing at work, I turned to my therapist, with whom I often spoke about how people treated me and my feelings of injustice and unfairness. One day, I noticed that my therapist was calling me "Megu" instead of "Meg." I was completely unaware of her calling me by my Japanese name until that day. At the same time, my therapy sessions helped me to explore counter-transference with my co-workers and patients. Instead of viewing them as trying to objectify me as an Asian, which made me hostile to them, I began to see them as reaching out and trying to relate. I started to make a conscious effort to address the elephant in the room by introducing myself with my Japanese name. Some people found my name difficult to pronounce and couldn't remember it because it wasn't as American as "Ann," "Jen," "Michelle," or "Nancy." So they associated it with an American cartoon, "Mr. Magoo." Sometime later, I found out from my adult patients that Mr. Magoo was "an old guy who couldn't see well, and always got into trouble," to which I thought, "He's almost blind, and I'm a 'color-blind therapist'. That's a perfect association!" Since then, whenever people had trouble with my name, I'd say, "You know, like *Mr. Magoo?*" Immediately, I'd see their eyes sparkle and an imaginary light bulb light up above their heads—ding-ding-ding!

When I finally accepted my name and that I was neither a White woman nor a White therapist, my interactions with my patients grew more natural, playful, and sincere. I decided to be honest and open with their questions. "Do you speak Chinese?" was answered with, "No, but I speak Japanese because I grew up in Japan." This paved the way for very interesting conversations and interactions. Some patients told me about how they used to take Asian language classes in college, how their best friends were from China, Japan, or South Korea, and how they enjoyed going to Chinese take-out restaurants because they were more affordable. Others talked about their lives being weighed down by illnesses, addictions, traumatic childhood memories, or broken and separated families. Responding to, "You live in Chinatown, don't you?" I would say, "No, I don't. But I used to go to a high school in Chinatown, and I love Chinese dim sum!" Some mentioned their Jewish heritage and said they didn't celebrate Christmas; instead, they went to Chinatown and ate at Chinese restaurants because they were always open. We talked about Asian food, which I found brought us closer and allowed us to learn more about each other. We also discussed their thoughts on Asian food being healthier, and their views on traditional Chinese medicine and how they wanted to try them because of the problems they had with western medication. To quote Acton (2001), "It is my position that is it unethical for the therapist to ignore my cultural background. By choosing to dismiss such an essential aspect of my life, the 'color-blind' therapist would not have all the vital components necessary to understand who I am" (pp. 111–112).

Art Therapy Group Examples

In my art therapy group sessions, some older patients talked about being in Okinawa during World War II. Their stories about war experiences were educational and I learned a lot about war history and their personal experiences in Japan, South Korea, and Vietnam. One day, I had two interns in my open art studio; one was from China, and the other from South Korea. Fifteen minutes after the group introduction during which everyone introduced themselves, a 73-year-old Black male patient, commented, out of the blue, that he had fought in the Vietnam War. I immediately glanced over at the interns, who looked visibly uncomfortable. As Lee (2005) said, "My greatest learning has come from situations in which I was willing to take risks, feel uncomfortable, and let go of safe, familiar, unquestioned beliefs" (p. 100). This was a situation I couldn't ignore. It was a chance to teach my patients and the students that racial comments, even when delivered innocuously, should be addressed immediately with more tact. I asked the patient, "May I ask you something? If you feel uncomfortable, let me know." He allowed me to proceed, and I said, "I have two Asian students in this group, and I'm from Japan. I found it interesting that you mentioned the Vietnam War with three Asian women present in this room. Would you like to comment on that?" He casually responded, "Oh, I have nothing against you, ladies. You seem so nice, and I like Asian people. I met the nicest people in Vietnam while I served." I said nothing to give him more time to add and elaborate. But very often, with patients whose thought processes aren't as fluid or logical, as is the case with this particular patient, conversations would abruptly end. Not much else was said and the session continued. Though the session remained superficial and awkward on some level, some tension was at least lifted from the air, and the interns felt more relaxed. At the same time, I asked others to chime in on how they felt about having three Asian women facilitate the group, their experiences in Asian countries, and to share any other memories and feelings related to their ethnic backgrounds. Many patients said, "I treat everyone the same way, regardless of their skin color. I'm not racist." Without explaining that it was not possible to really treat everyone the same way without comprehending their race and culture, I thanked them for their contribution. I was there to listen to their opinions, not to lecture them. This session was a personal achievement for me. By raising the issue of race and ethnicity in my session, I proved that I was not afraid of addressing the issue of race.

Some of my patients were naturally curious about Asian writings. They often asked, "Can you write Chinese?" I would reply, "We have a similar writing system that we borrowed from China. I can read some Chinese writing, though their pronunciations are different." Then I would ask them, "Would you like to learn to write Japanese characters?" So I created a Japanese calligraphy group, which was an interactive activity that promoted attentiveness, patience, and a sense of achievement. They would ask me to write their names in Japanese, not only in Chinese characters but also in Hiragana and Katakana. We have three different writing systems or alphabets in Japan: Hiragana, Katakana, and Kanji. Kanji is adopted from Chinese writing that requires many years of training. It is most common to start from Hiragana when Japanese people first learn to write. However, many patients were attracted Kanji and that's they often wish to write.

I encouraged them to practice the writings on their own time. I also provided Sumi, Japanese ink. My patients decorated their names, which they gifted to their family and staff members. While working with younger adults, they taught me the art of bubble letters and tag names. I also introduced Sumi to older adults, and some became excited to talk about their experiences having tattoo in Kanji. Others were intimidated because they'd never used Sumi before. Nevertheless, the end drawings were still organic and fluid. They even used their artwork as wrapping papers for small gifts or to wrap wine bottles. Here are some of the examples that I have made for my patients (Figures 2.1–2.4).

One of the most amusing things that happened with adult patients was when they brought along Origami books and instructions and asked me to make them. Because I never learned Origami through instruction books, I found having to refer to instructions to be counterproductive. One time, while trying to make an Origami giraffe, I lost my patience and gave up, throwing the attempted giraffe aside. Laughter broke out across the group, and they insisted, "But you are Japanese!" I said, "I can't do it! I just can't." That shattered the patients' stereotypical views of not only the Japanese being masters of Origami but also therapists who should be leading by example instead of discouraging patients by giving up on a task. At that moment, the patient-therapist barrier dissolved and we

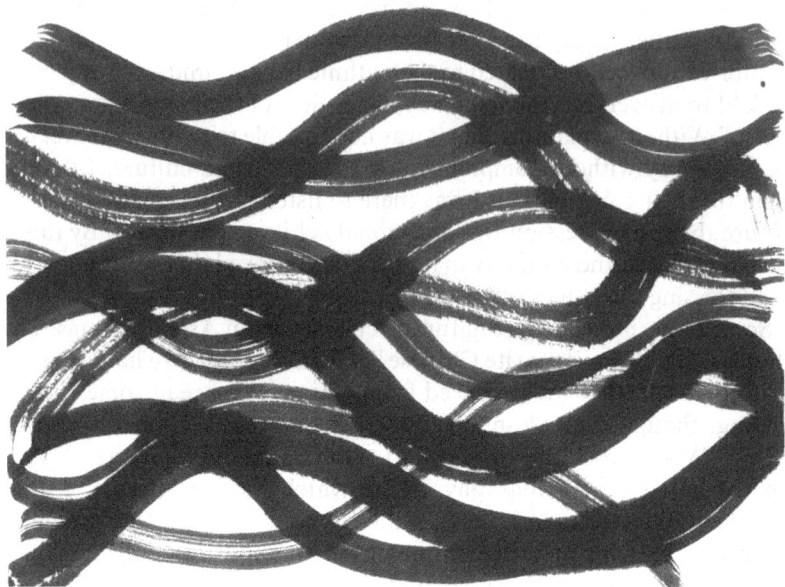

Figure 2.1 Sumi Ink example by Megu Kitazawa.

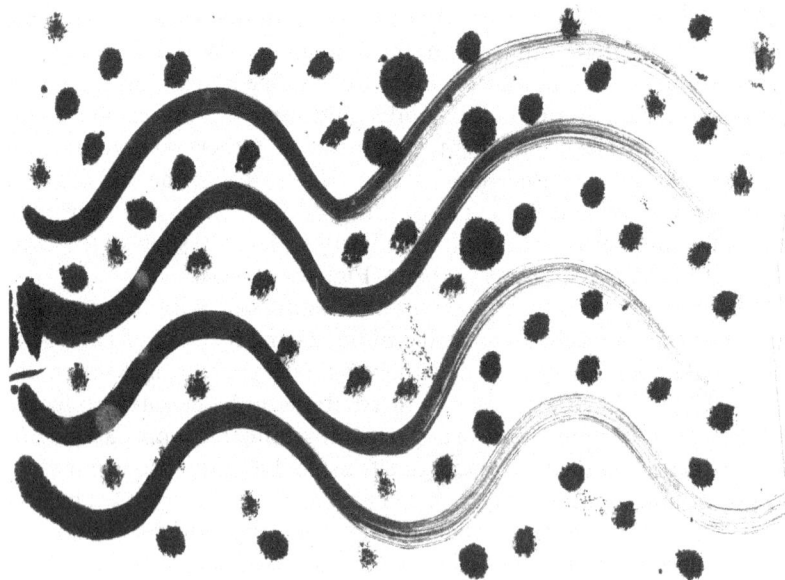

Figure 2.2 Sumi Ink example by Megu Kitazawa.

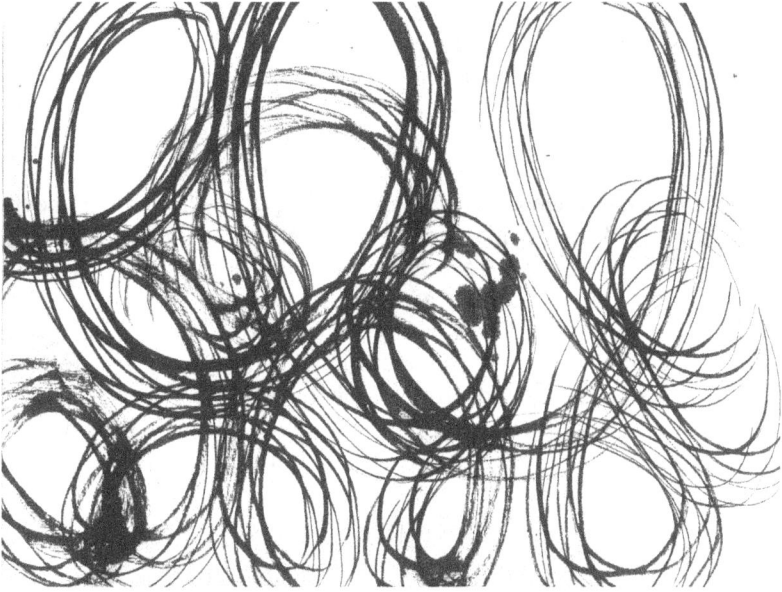

Figure 2.3 Sumi Ink example by Megu Kitazawa.

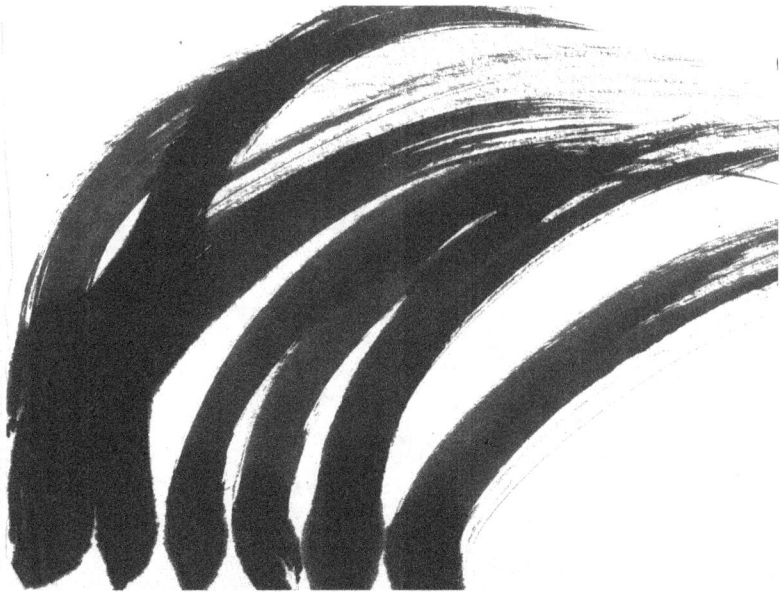

Figure 2.4 Sumi Ink example by Megu Kitazawa.

became less of patients and art therapists and more of human beings who were all just trying to figure things out.

Other times, I had male patients who were fascinated with Geishas, a few of whom wanted to draw a portrait of me. Since it was an open art studio, I was moving around to help other patients. They would tell me, "Stop moving," "Move to the right," "No, look this way." As their subject of drawing, I was obliged to do as they asked. As a result, they felt like they were being heard and people were paying attention to them. Incidentally, most of their finished portraits ended up as gifts to me, which I humbly accepted and praised their astute observations. I remained neutral about their drawings and held back on interpreting and analyzing them too deeply, including any possible erotic transference. Some even said, "I thought Asian people looked the same, but I realized that wasn't true when I was drawing you." Images in Figures 2.5–2.8 are all drawn by my former adult patients in psychiatric inpatient units.

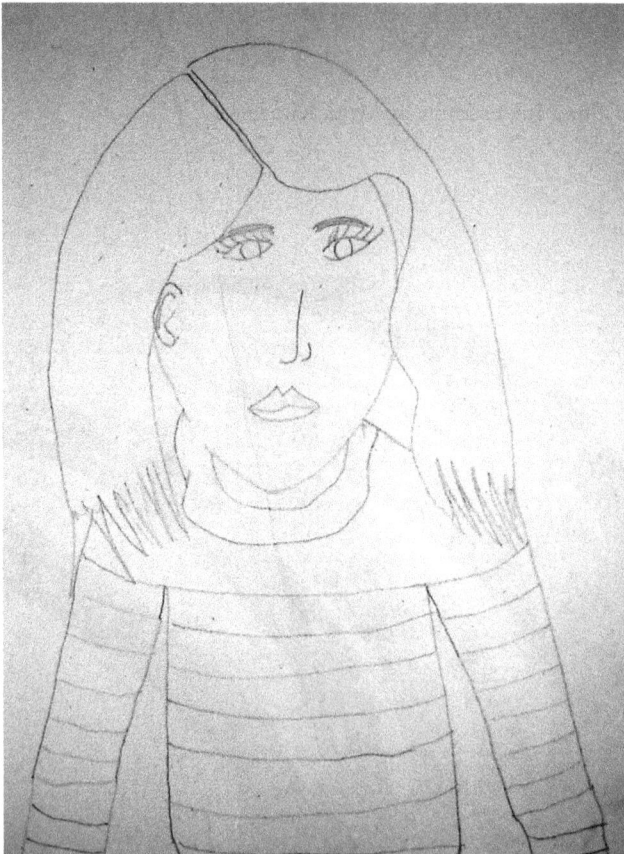

Figure 2.5 Portrait of Megu by an adult patient in a NYC psychiatric hospital.

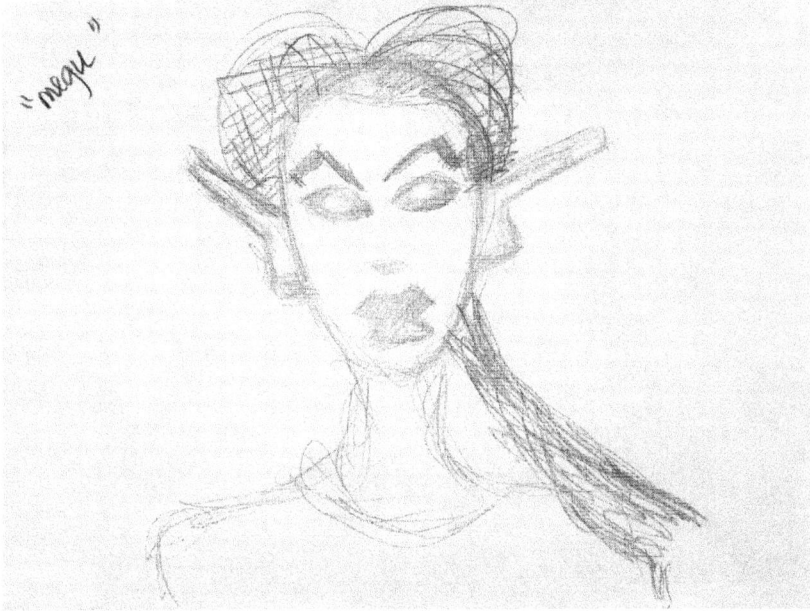

Figure 2.6 Portrait of Megu by an adult patient in a NYC psychiatric hospital.

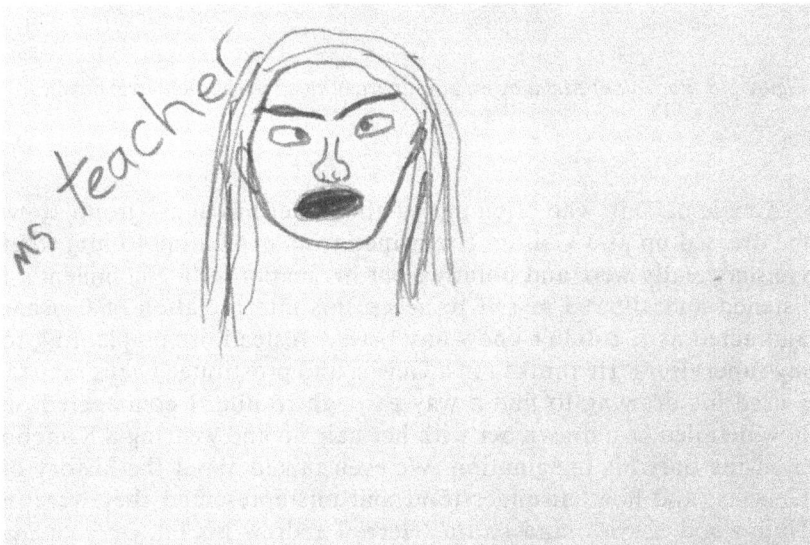

Figure 2.7 Portrait of Megu by an adult patient in a NYC psychiatric hospital.

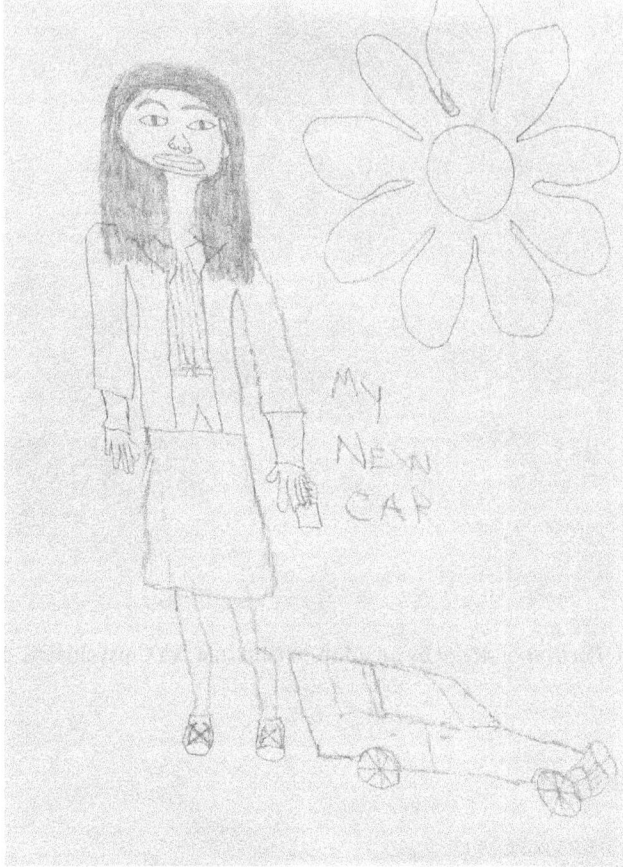

Figure 2.8 Portrait of Megu by an adult patient in a NYC psychiatric hospital.

A male patient, who often talked about Geishas in my group, drew me dressed up as a Geisha. I refrained from explaining to him what Geishas really were and pointing out his inappropriate comments. I listened and allowed myself to accept his interpretation of Geishas and acted as if I didn't know any better. Instead of complaining to my supervisor, "He thinks I'm a Geisha and prostitute! That's racist," I used his drawing to find a way through to him. I commented on how detailed he'd drawn her with her hair up and wearing a Kimono by using only his imagination. We even talked about the history of Geishas, and how misunderstood and misrepresented they were in Hollywood movies, and so on. Here, I redrew his image from my memory (Figure 2.9).

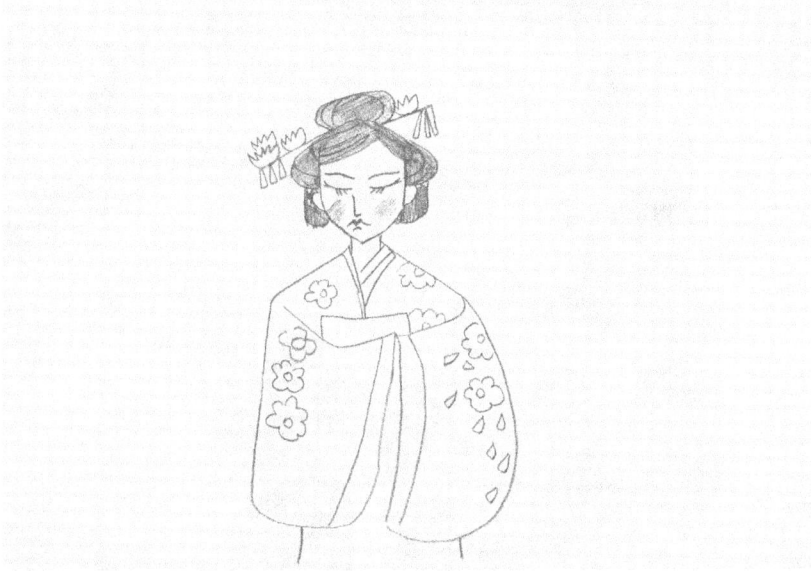

Figure 2.9 A patient's Geisha image by Megu Kitazawa drawn from her memory.

My change in approach led to interactions that were eye-openings for me. I had expected them to treat people differently based on their racial and cultural backgrounds. But because most had never had such interactions with a Japanese person, they simply weren't conscious about doing so. Despite having lived in NYC their entire lives, these patients never had the opportunity to have proper and meaningful conversations with a Japanese woman. For many of them, their sessions with me were their first interaction with an Asian person. Just recently in January 2020, I snapped this picture in my neighborhood. This young Asian woman dressed in a Kimono and wearing traditional Geisha makeup gazes lustfully after its viewers to lure it into the world of Japan. Because it's based on the general and stereotypical association and fascination with Japan, it's relatable and it does a great job at catching people's attention. Whereas before when such posters would stir up feelings of unease in me and make me feel objectified, I was now humored by it, and I realized I was now in a place where I was able to find such stereotypes amusing and say to myself: It is not about me (Figure 2.10).

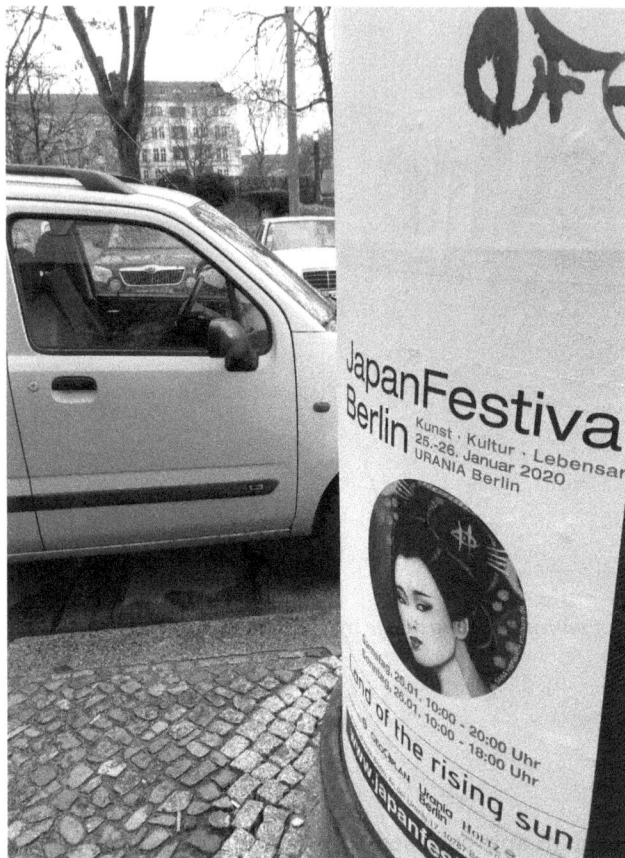

Figure 2.10 Japan festival poster in Berlin. Photograph taken by Megu Kitazawa.

Conclusion

Through my interactions with my patients, I stumbled upon my own biases of being an "Americanized" and "non-White" woman who only imitated the behaviors and mannerisms of White women. I realized that I needed only to accept that I wasn't White to have honest, open, and safe discussions with my patients that could spontaneously lead to self-reflection and insights. And I have learned a great deal about being an art therapist that I carry with me even to this day. I might have taken steps that can be viewed as anti-analytic and none-art-therapy-like along the way. Those interventions, verbal or visual, were trial and error. But surprisingly, most of the encounters turned out not only to be positive, but also helped to deepen and enrich my relationships with my patients. As therapists, we are privileged to listen to their stories (or even lies and frustrations) that our patients may feel uncomfortable sharing even with their closest friends or family members. I found some of Lee's (2005) advice on therapists as "compassionate witness to clients of color" (p. 113) to be very helpful. Larry Jin Lee is a Chinese American social worker in San Francisco. Below are some of Lee's (2005) extracts:

> Get out of the way. Don't interrupt. It is not about you—don't make it about you.
>
> Practice mindfully observing your reactions rather than rushing in to fix the client's problem.
>
> Practice and embrace not knowing. This will create more space for the client's experience to be visible.
>
> When in doubt, ask permission. Don't assume trust exists.
>
> Explore and become aware of the masks you have had to wear to function in the world. (p. 113)

I visited Japan for the first time in eight years in April 2019. Though I hadn't lived there for over 30 years, my behaviors and mannerism very naturally and instinctively became more Japanese when I was there. I was more conscious around commuters to avoid disturbing their personal spaces and was more mindful of what others thought of me when chatting too loudly with my mother in public. "Excuse me" and "I am so sorry" rolled off my tongue very naturally in the crowded streets of Tokyo, just as bows did in restaurants and stores. I realized that I would never feel at "home" in either Japan or the United States. But I'm now aware of the different masks I wear when I'm in one place or another. And that's not a bad thing.

References

Acton, D. (2001). The "color blind" therapist. *Art Therapy: Journal of the American Art Therapy Association*, *18*(2), 109–112. http://dx.doi.org/10.1080/07421656.20 01.10129749

Afshar, D. (2017). *15 Stereotypes all Japanese people hate*. The culture trip. Retrieved from https://theculturetrip.com/asia/japan/articles/15-stereotypes-all-japanese-people-hate/

Awais, Y. J., & Yali, A. M. (2015). Efforts in increasing racial and ethnic diversity in the field of art therapy. *Art Therapy: Journal of the American Art Therapy Association*, *32*(3), 112–119. https://doi.org/10.1080/07421656.2015.1060842

Doby-Copeland, C. (2006). Cultural diversity curriculum design: An art therapist's perspective. *Art Therapy: Journal of the American Art Therapy Association*, *23*(4), 172–180. http://dx.doi.org/10.1080/07421656.2006.10129330

Elkins, D. E., & Deaver, S. P. (2015). American art therapy association, Inc.: 2013 membership survey report. *Art Therapy: Journal of the American Art Therapy Association*, *32*(2), 60–69.

George, J., Brooke, D.G., & Blackwell, M. (2005). Three voices on multiculturalism in the art therapy classroom. *Art Therapy: Journal of the American Art Therapy Association, 22*(3), 132–138. http://doi.org/10.1080/07421656.2005.10129492

Immigrant generations. (n.d.) In *Wikipedia*. Retrieved March 22, 2020, from https://en.wikipedia.org/wiki/immigrant_generations

Lee, L. J. (2005). Taking off the mask: Breaking the silence—the art of naming racism in the therapy room. In M. Rastogi & E. Wieling (Eds.), *Voices of color: First-person accounts of ethnic minority therapists* (pp. 91–115). Sage Publications.

3 Returning to the Sacred Circle, Immigrant and Indigenous Allies

A Heuristic Perspective

Sheba Sheikhai

Introduction

This chapter will explore my experience as a first generation, Asian-American art therapist processing my multi-cultural identity while in graduate school and working cross-culturally with the Urban Native American community. By sharing a heuristic review of my anecdotes, artworks, and writings, I hope to illuminate parallels between Eastern and Western cultures, and journey through the intersectionality of Immigrant and Indigenous experiences. In addition, I will demonstrate how grounding in Joan Kellogg's Great Round theory and holistic healing models can combat colonizing mentality as well as facilitate insights for cultural identity integration.

Sacred Circle

A perennial icon of humanity, the symbol of the circle has been regarded as an important metaphysical concept and tool for shamanistic and ritual practices, designating a space that is to be considered sacred or protected. From my North East Indian heritage, I know this symbol in the form of the Tibetan sand mandala. The sacred artwork is created in colorful sand by Buddhist monks and is eventually brushed away to demonstrate the temporary nature of all things. The intricate designs can symbolize the entirety of the Universe, holding space for a deity, or a path to human enlightenment.

From my work within the Urban Native community, I've learned that the sacred circle lives at the core of Native American values and spirituality. Represented at times by the four-quadrant Medicine Wheel, it offers a holistic healing model that can symbolize an interconnected system of teachings relating to the seasons, natural elements and realms of human existence—physical, emotional, mental, and spiritual. However, Natives' overall understanding of the Sacred Hoop can go beyond the four corners or realms. In the words of my mentor, Dustin Tyee Richardson, a descendant of the Blackfeet tribe, "It is the sacred center that dwells within each of us. It is Creator and the heart of the Universe. It is a reminder that we are part of the sacred and that all of living existence draws consciousness in us with every heartbeat."

In art therapy, we can relate this shared human consciousness to Carl Jung's mandala reflections in *The Red Book* (Jung, 2009) and his belief in archetypal models as unconscious human psychological inheritance. We can further apply an archetypal framework to stages of life span development through Joan Kellogg's theory of the Archetypal Stages of the Great Round of Mandala. This theory offers a system for identifying archetypes as phases of consciousness which can be used to track processes ranging "from the evolution of man, to the development of an idea, to the stages of a relationship" (Takei, 2015).

When looking at traditional motifs of the Tibetan mandala and the Native Medicine Wheel through the lens of the Great Round, we can see that both might capture the essence of Stage 7: "Squaring the Circle" (Figure 3.1). At this stage, there is an archetypal emphasis on wholeness,

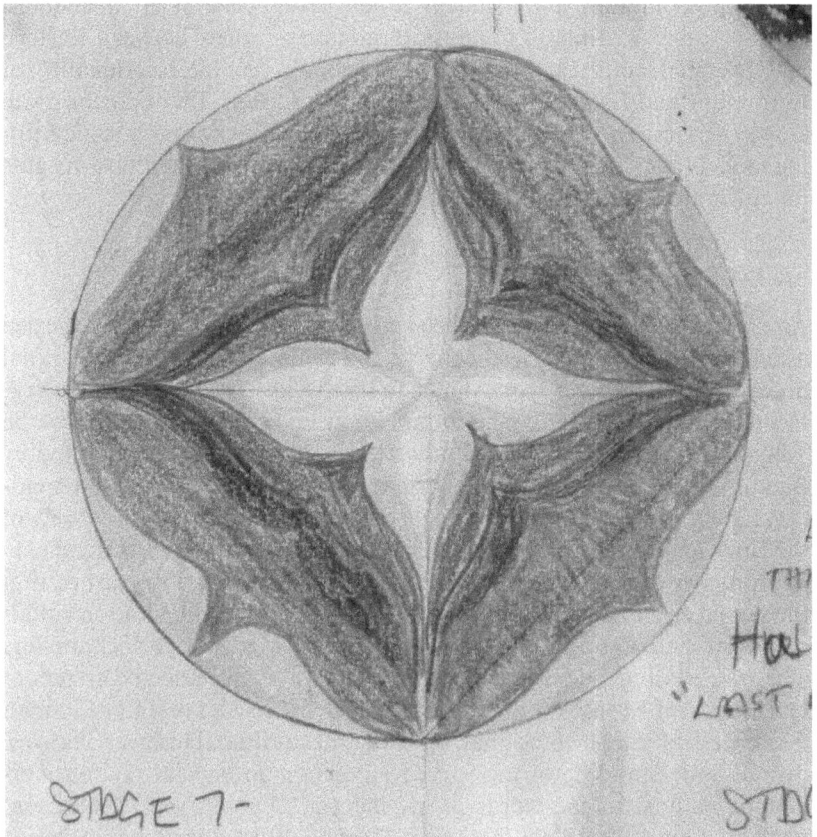

Figure 3.1 Stage 7: Squaring the Circle by Sheba Sheikhai.

integration and perfect balance between opposites. Jung remarked, "the 'squaring of the circle' is one of the many archetypal motifs which form the basic patterns of our dreams and fantasies" (Tokyo: Kodansha, 1983). When noticing this synergy between Eastern and Western cultures, I was intrigued by the shared desire to connect with a whole greater than the sum of its parts, and how this human propensity has the power to transcend geographic, linguistic, and cultural barriers.

Home Salty Home

Prior to entering graduate school in 2017, I attempted to connect with my North East Indian and Buddhist roots by visiting my mother's family in Kalimpong, West Bengal. My father is native to Iran and though I have begged to visit, all too often his response is: "it is not safe to go right now." It's been over 30 years since he has been back to his home country.

I greatly anticipated my voyage to India as a "coming home" that I've waited for my whole life thus far. I imagined it would be filled with long meditative walks, views of the sacred Himalayas, visits to temples in the foothills, and most importantly, my Ama's (grandmother's) homemade aloo parathas and chana dal. Unfortunately, I never made it to my grandparents' house. During the time I was in India, there was a travel ban in the North East region due to considerable political and civil unrest between the local peoples of the foothills, Indian Gurkhas, and the West Bengal government. The peoples of Kalimpong and neighboring Darjeeling have long been exploited for their fertile lands and agriculture, and some have been calling for a separate Gorkhaland nation state since the 1980s. My mother says this conflict had started long before she was born. I ended up staying in the city of Kolkata with my aunts and uncles for the remainder of the trip. My aunt relayed the news of local riots, police violence, and arson in the foothills. Most salient was a news photograph that revealed their hometown center in flames. The center housed a clock tower that my great grandfather had maintained in his work as a repair technician. When I shared this news with my mother, she said she didn't want to think about it as it made her too sad. My heart broke for her, for myself, and our relatives. I wrote a brief phrase in my journal in response to the image: "home salty home," for the whole experience offered a sharp taste of reality rather than the sweet homecoming I had imagined. I started to see that for many there may never be a way back, therefore we must find a way forward.

Chameleon

In graduate school, when we began to learn about the Great Round theory, we were guided in meditation, reflecting on "how am I doing right now?" After the exercise, I created this mandala based off of an image

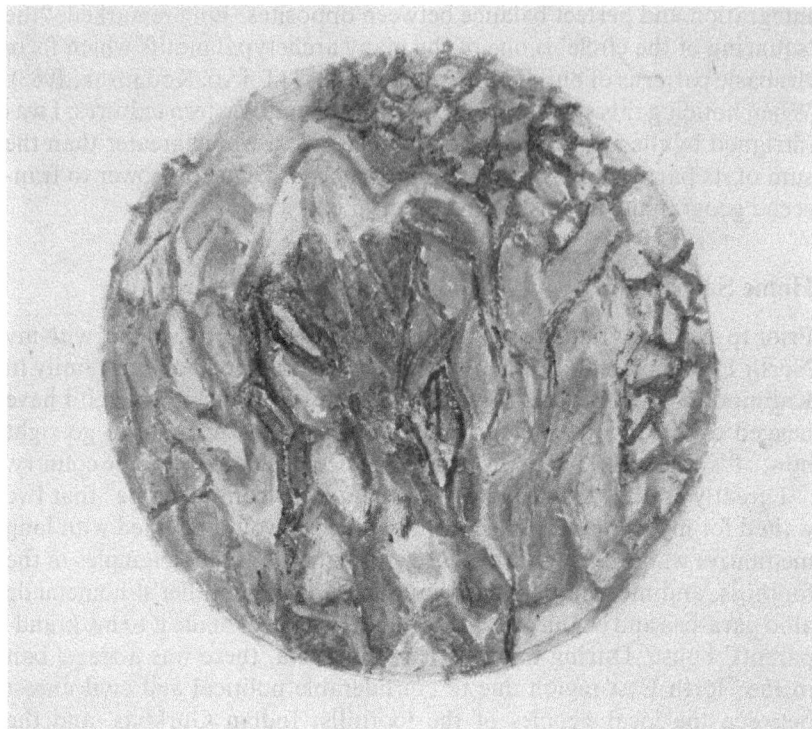

Figure 3.2 Chameleon, Stage 11: Fragmentation by Sheba Sheikhai.

that came to mind (Figure 3.2). I envisioned a chameleon, always shifting in shape and color. I imagined what it might look like to zoom in with a microscope to see the details of its skin, to really know what drives its pretty colors.

In processing the mandala through the Great Round lens, I was able to identify that at this point, I was at Stage 11: "Fragmentation." At this stage there can be a sense of release, chaos v. shattering, and decomposition. In retrospect, the metaphor of the chameleon is a fitting description for how I often see myself—adapting to different people and environments, changing colors, and character to blend in. The theme of fragmentation also made sense as my ego-identity seemed to be coming apart, in order to embark on my subsequent journey into new self-awareness and cross-cultural insights.

Water Is Life

I was introduced to contemporary Native American issues from attending a talk regarding the Dakota Access Pipeline water crisis. At this time, I was in the first year of my graduate program and was volunteering at an aquaponics greenhouse. The panel consisted of Native nonprofit leaders, lawyers, and environment activists who spoke to the concept of "Mni Wiconi: Water is Life," and the duty the Indigenous Peoples of the area felt to protect the life-giving waters for their communities. They shared information about Standing Rock tribal members conducting peaceful protests that had been met with police brutality and demolition of sacred grounds. I was struck by the irony of how police used water cannons as riot control, using it against the very people who honored the element as a life-giving force.

I was shocked hearing some of these issues for the first time, wondering how this news of ongoing oppression seemed so sheltered. I was impressed by the panelists and how Natives of today are so enthusiastically involved in political justice. I became intrigued by a statement one of the panelists made, referring to the upholding of dominant narratives in our society as a "colonization of the mind." The phrase rang through my ears with haunting. The panel discussed how in operating from a colonizing mentality, we imply that we have a right to exercise dominion over natural resources, and that minority ethnic groups should assimilate to the majority in power. In recognizing this phenomenon, it seemed like my concept of America and what it meant to be "American" had shifted, now distinguishing that my own truth too, had been stirring in the shadow of this mindset.

The discussion was closed with a Lakota prayer and drum song. It was when I heard the sound of the drum and cries in the prayer that my heart began to beat with conviction. My own quiet song made a lump in my throat and it seemed as if the sacred waters flowed right into me, filling my eyes and soul with clarity and resonance. This experience was so impactful that it inspired my thesis research about the behavioral health of Urban Natives which segued into my current art therapy work with this community.

Duran (2006) writes of colonizing as a "dehumanizing activity" and that when the counseling profession "validates empirically tested therapies only from a Western logical positivistic paradigm, we engage in Western supremacy disguised as perceived scientific objectivity" (p. 14). This prejudice can be "a very subtle and clever neo-colonialism that will further alienate people and groups" and "decolonizing does not apply only to Native People or other people of color who have been colonized" (p. 14) suggesting that mainstream Westerners may too benefit from decolonizing consumer-focused processes that have been imposed on them.

The following mandala was created in processing my connection to water and the notion of "Higher Power" (Figure 3.3). When looking at the formal features, we can see there is a balance between humanity and this natural element. The water is depicted in color, while the hand is a simple line drawing, which seems to emphasize the water's dynamic

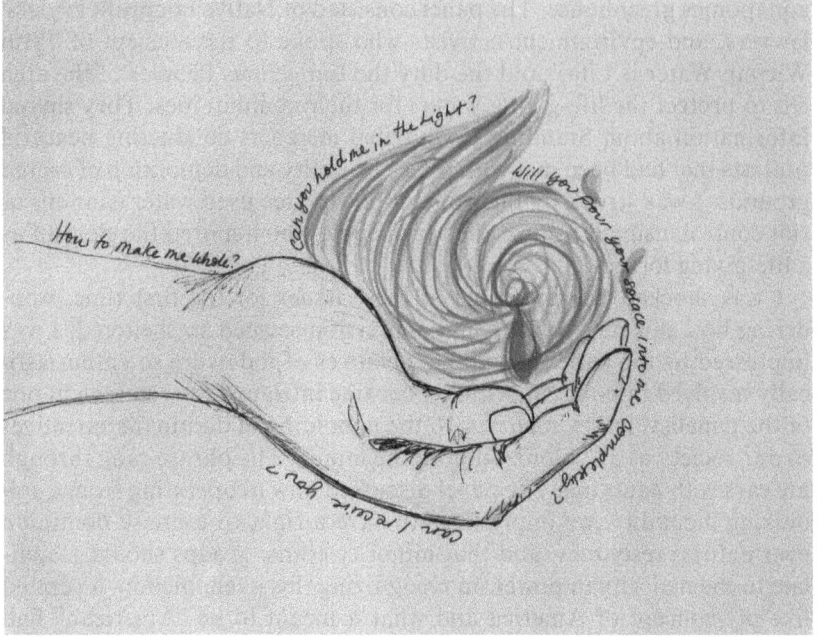

Figure 3.3 Mni Wiconi, Stage 3: Labyrinth/Spiral by Sheba Sheikhai.

and animating influence. However, the water is also contained within the hand, somewhat cultivated and kept. From the questions posed in my writings: "How to make me whole? Will you pour your solace into me completely?" It is evident that there is a longing for comfort, fulfillment, and wholeness. While the question of "Can I receive you?" might highlight the uncertainty in my ability to relate to, or learn from this source. In reference to the Great Round, this mandala might represent Stage 3: "Labyrinth/Spiral," concerned with focus, calling, excitement v. anxiety, and fetal development.

History and Hope

I created this piece in my graduate program's cultural diversity class, depicting efforts to hold two truths of my identity in balance—values of a collectivist immigrant home life and the individualism of U.S. society (Figure 3.4). In the art making process, it was difficult for me to know what images would represent my "American" identity. The symbols I chose appeared a bit generic to me. However, an element of continuity seems to be represented by the Mala prayer beads wrapped around both

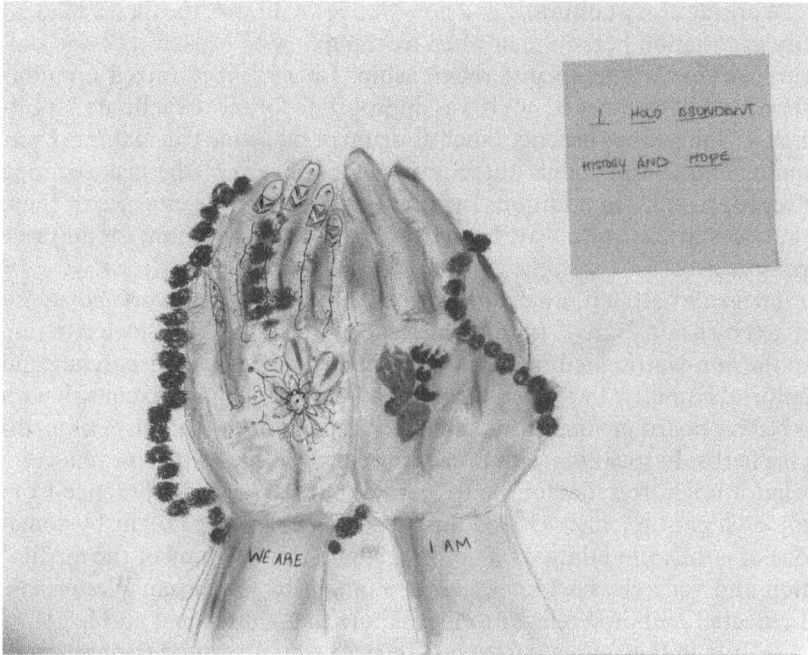

Figure 3.4 Duality by Sheba Sheikhai.

hands. I added the caption: "I hold abundant history and hope." It felt at times destabilizing to not fully be able to root in one world or the other; however, I found grounding in development of my own integrative faith and rituals.

Later in my work with Urban Native clients, the concept of "identity negotiation" and "walking two paths" manifested when grappling with conflict between one's Native and non-Native identities, or a two spirit identity. This seemed to identify a common struggle among both Natives and Immigrants. For myself and my clients, I learned that cultivating the capacity to accept two seemingly opposing truths in balance and reframing this unique perspective as a strength can help reconcile distress with contradiction. We can refer to this reframing mechanism as "hybrid" thinking, which Duran (2006) refers to as a post-colonial concept that recognizes "there can be two or more ways of knowing and this can be a harmonious process" (p. 14). Duran further applies this concept to transcend hierarchical notions of "cross-cultural" or "cultural sensitivity" through the term, "epistemological hybridism," which honors and accepts the worldviews of a person or group as a valid and core truth (p. 14).

Working cross-culturally as a non-Native facilitator, the theme of identity negotiation perpetuated when learning how to broach race and culture within the therapeutic relationship. I experienced mixed opinions from staff of whether or not it was appropriate for me to facilitate "traditional" Indigenous practices such as drum or medicine bag making. I was quite nervous to conduct these groups for concern of the task seeming "appropriated." In addition, I learned that every tribe engages in these practices in their own way. I worried, "how could I account for all these perspectives?"

I began by attending a drum and medicine bag making workshop facilitated by a non-Native. In this experience I took note of my own reaction to the non-Native facilitator and their ability to model transparency and cultural humility. I was then recommended by my mentor to consult with a Native board member who had experience in traditional uses of medicine herbs. In speaking with him of my concerns, he helped me reflect on what it might feel like for me to learn about a traditional practice from my own culture, such as Buddhist teachings or yoga, taught by someone of a different ethnicity. I could relate to this as many of the meditation and yoga classes I do attend are taught by Caucasian Westerners. I reflected on how I related to instructors that I respected and felt were authentic in their practice, versus the ones who presented themselves as "all-knowing" or imposed a one-sided perspective. By noticing how I experienced forms of this phenomenon myself, it helped dispel hierarchical assumptions and allowed me to empathize with my clients on a more mutual level.

What ultimately transpired from this process was the understanding of the importance of self-reflection and holding people in conversation. It is called identity negotiation for a reason—to communicate about one another's expectations, self-perceptions, and perceptions of others. Leaning into these discussions with clients has helped me to realize that if I present a cultural-based task with transparency of who I am, and what I know and do not know, it enables both clients and staff to collaborate in sharing their own viewpoints, concerns, and feedback on how they relate to me as a facilitator. It is in these mutual, conversational spaces that both my clients and myself have the opportunity to affirm our own cultures and explore varying levels of identification with "traditional" or "contemporary" practices.

Processing this concept in practicum supervision, I created this mandala (Figure 3.5). To me, it represents corresponding balance, reflection, and a respectful dynamic, similar with Yin and Yang energies, that can be maintained by holding one another in conversation. Through a Great Round lens, this image in Figure 3.5 may fall into Stage 6: "Dragon Fight," concerned with opposites, shadow, balance v. conflict, and adolescence.

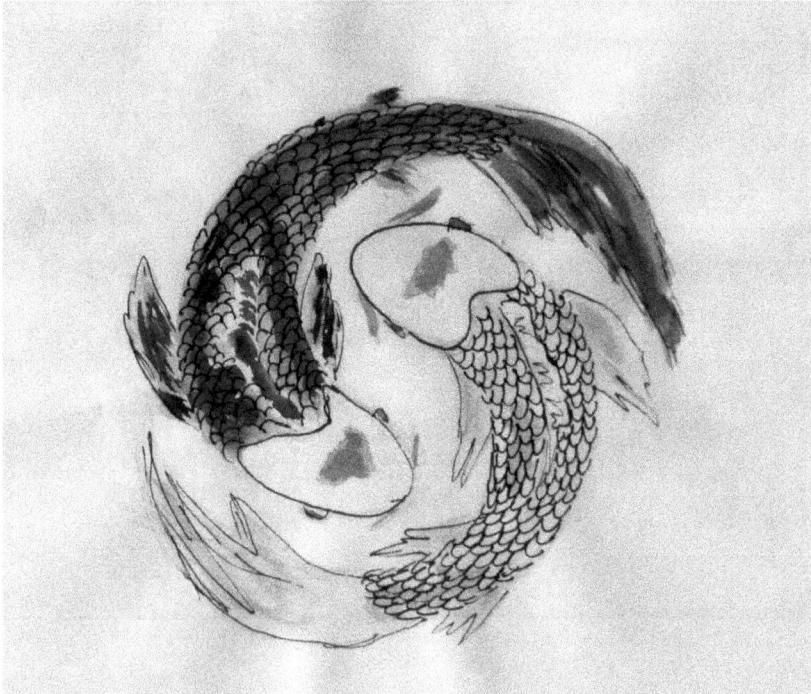

Figure 3.5 Negotiation, Stage 6: Dragon Fight by Sheba Sheikhai.

Bad American, Good Foreigner

In my ethics class, we were asked to take implicit association tests (IATs) to better understand our own biases and perspectives. I took two tests. The first explored social bias which yielded an automatic association for "American" with "White America," and "Foreign" with "Native American." The second test explored self-esteem, and suggested that I strongly identify myself more with "good" than "bad."

Considering these two findings in conjunction, I thought about my own ethnicity and experience growing up as a first-generation American, born to immigrant parents from India and Iran. I realized that my collectivist home life was highly contrasted to the more individualistic ideals I was being taught through school and socializing. However, having one foot in each culture seemed to separate me from feeling fully accepted or comfortable in either. My family chose not to pass down their languages in efforts for me to better assimilate, however, this left me disconnected from a vital part of my heritage by way of communication barrier. My elders often struggled to understand my "Americanized" ways and slang, while at school I was bullied and discriminated for being "brown" and having a "foreign" accent.

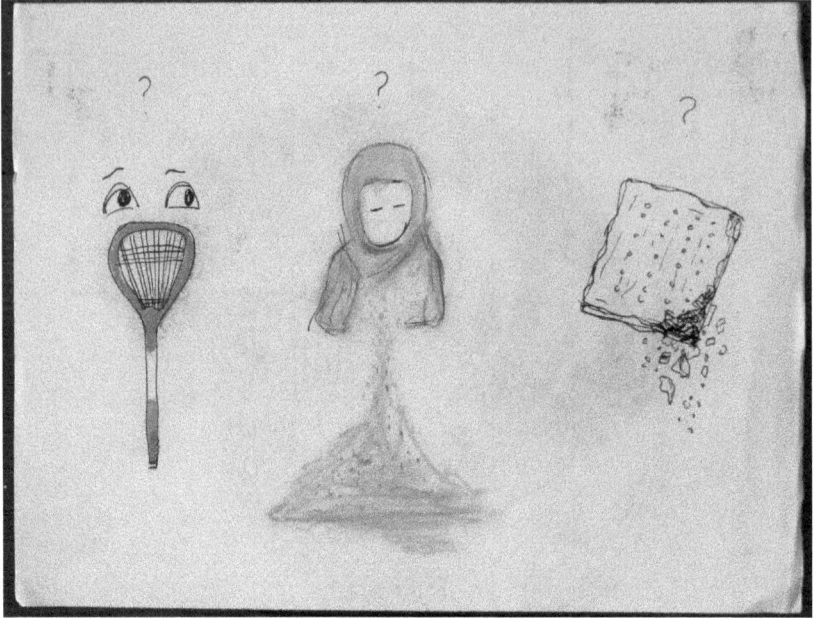

Figure 3.6 Diversity Continuum by Sheba Sheikhai.

I realized these experiences have caused me to think of myself on a contin-uum of "good" and "bad" depending on the environment and other people's perceptions of me. For some, I might seem "White washed" for a person of color, and this may be comforting, but for others it might be disappointing.

The artwork in Figure 3.6 was made in reflection of this continuum. The images represent times that I was called derogatory slurs of "foreigner," "sand nigger," and "cracker." I could see how each could apply to me; how-ever, what I found most interesting is that these were such diverse interpreta-tions of who I am, regardless of my actual race or cultural background. The recognition of this continuum was both concerning and freeing for me, in that I saw how discrimination can be so superficial while also learning that other's interpretations of me ultimately don't dictate who I am.

Self-Portrait

I became drawn to the Urban Native American community and ways of life as I recognized similarities between my parent's immigrant experience and the experience of the Indigenous Peoples of America. Commonalities of displacement, discrimination, loss of culture, and equity all seem to par-allel in the pain and loss incurred from subjugation by dominant, colonial narratives. However, as a cross-cultural art therapist, I must maintain a cau-tious awareness of my own bias toward "White America" and how this can potentially inhibit me from having compassion for dominant attitudes or ethnicities. This knowledge is important when working with Urban Natives as due to interracial mingling, many can present and identify as Caucasian.

Even for these clients, and those who identify more with Native American or mixed-minority race, it has been interesting to see how being a person of color has benefitted me in building rapport. Some clients even assume that I am Native American. However, when I reveal that I am an Immigrant and speak of my own Asian-indigenous mountain roots, the responses are mixed but overall filled with curiosity and to my surprise, share the acknowledgment of our cultural parallels. That said, I am not exempt from the process of building mutual trust and respect in order to be "invited in" to engage personal or sacred topics. As within any therapeutic relationship, I've learned that nurturing authentic connections are key to maintaining cultural competence and humility.

The self-portrait in Figure 3.7 was created in response to the IAT exercise. It explores my cultural identity, self-perspective, and growing awareness

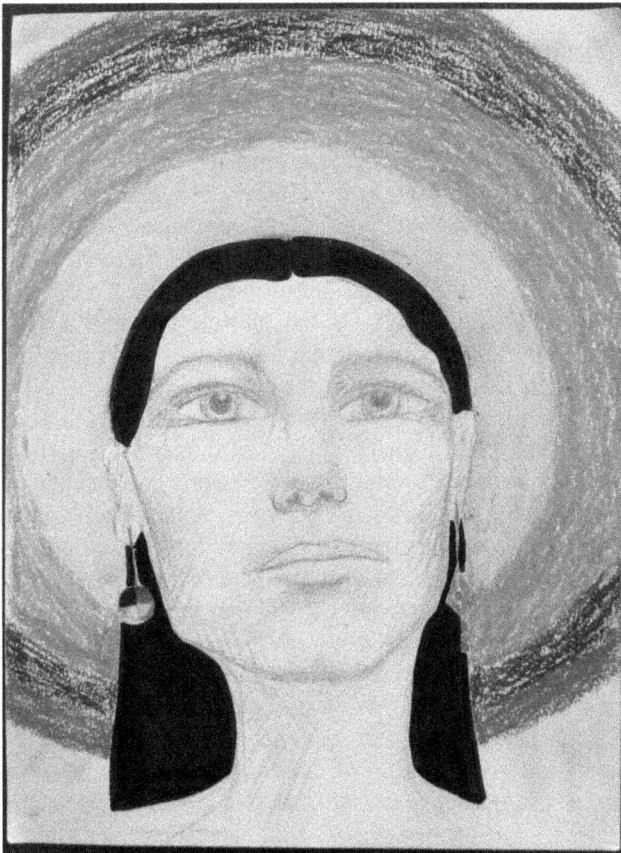

Figure 3.7 Self-Portrait, Stage 5: Target by Sheba Sheikhai.

of a potential bias against "White American" culture. The earrings symbolize cultural parallels between my North East Indian heritage with that of Western Native America as they hold synonymously rich histories of artistry, stonework, and beadwork. The Medicine Wheel on the left represents Native spirituality and grounding in elements, and the earring to the right represents prominent use of coral and turquoise in Tibetan handicraft. I've grown to collect and appreciate jewelry from around the world, regarding them as aesthetic totems for the diversity of humanity. The concentric rings of yellow, brown, red, and white, abstract skin tones and emulate new circles of consciousness. Through a Great Round lens, we can see that the background's archetypal image is present in Stage 5: "Target," concerned with power, boundaries v. defenses, and childhood. This is a significant theme in maintaining awareness of racial bias and over-identification. In processing this piece, I realize I had unconsciously portrayed my own image as a black and white sketch, perhaps still perceiving myself as somewhat unfinished and becoming.

Cultural Trauma and Resiliency

Throughout my graduate program and work with Urban Native community, I've had the privilege of reflecting on my experience as being a multi-cultural person of color, and am learning how to embrace and take ownership of these parts of my identity, especially in the field of art therapy. This may have contributed to the perspective of seeing myself as "good" even learning to appreciate and accept a struggle with my own mental health within the contexts of cultural trauma.

Wiechelt et al. (2020) emphasize that "culture provides a structure and context in which members can define themselves and make meaning of the events in their lives as well as in the collective. Cultures often contain a paradigm as to how the world operates in relation to a divine force" (p. 172). They note that a disintegration of culture can be traumatic as it removes a vital support system of which both individuals and groups can otherwise rely on to organize their lives, sense of self and other, and ability to cope with external stressors. They further comment, that "as with PTSD, the experience of the event in and of itself is not traumatic; the interpretation and meaning that is attached to the event by a given culture influences whether or not it becomes traumatic for the culture" (p. 173).

Intergenerational transfer of trauma and post-traumatic stress are associated with increased rates of depression, drug use, and drug addiction (Martin & Shaw, 2017). For Natives, there is now an understanding "that alcoholism is a symptom of more deeply embedded wounds from the trauma of oppressive genocidal behaviors and policies caused from dominant Euro-American society" that have been persistently passed down from generation to generation (Coyhis & Simonelli, 2008). I've witnessed these inherited occurrences among the Urban Native community and within my own Asian-immigrant family. A disruption from cultural origins and practices through displacement, acculturation difficulties, and generational desertion has resulted in the perpetuation of impoverished and self-defeating cultural narratives. In efforts to heal and build resilience within Indigenous communities, a "return to culture" healing-centered model is a leading approach in the Wellbriety Movement of Native substance use recovery.

Through cross-cultural engagement, I've personally experienced the benefits of applying a "return to culture" model for Immigrant wellness, particularly from a background of collectivist values. Gaining a sense of self-esteem and self-knowledge from connecting with my own heritage and racial identity, as well as exploring others, has been an important part of both my personal and professional growth. This is reflected in my final artwork (Figure 3.8). The efficacy of this cultural-based healing approach is significant for holistic integration, as it can account for multiple levels of being and knowing, particularly connecting on a soul and spiritual level to something greater than oneself. By developing a relationship with a the Divine through cross-cultural engagement with multiple environments, peoples, and facets within ourselves, we have the opportunity to restructure and restore our cultural narratives, which in turn, can fortify societal relations as a whole. It is through a collective and archetypal awareness that we can call upon our ancestors, relatives,

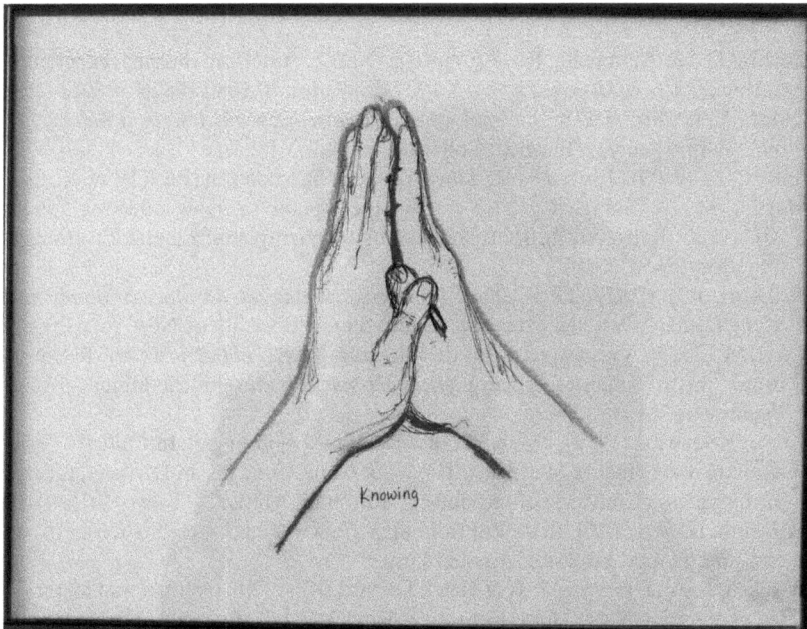

Figure 3.8 Knowing by Sheba Sheikhai.

and allies to nurture the roots of our existence, providing the foundations of resiliency and post-traumatic growth.

Conclusion

Overall, by uniquely empathizing with my diverse Native American clients and co-workers, I've learned how to embrace my own multi-cultural immigrant roots. This pivotal understanding has driven my purpose in advocating for marginalized peoples and communities in the field of art therapy. By returning to and grounding in the sacred circle, I feel that I am honoring my Asian ancestors and American kin. Processing my identity development through the Great Round theory, I've garnered holistic insights and perspective on cultural wellness. This continues to support and guide my cross-cultural interests and moral commitments as an art therapist of color.

In the words of Black Elk, an Oglala Sioux holy man, "Even the seasons form a great circle in their changing, and always come back again to where they were. The life of man is a circle from childhood to childhood, and so it is in everything where power moves" (Neihardt [1932] 2008). In order to heal and restore balance within our societies, it is vital for us to uphold the lost voices, faces, and places of all those whose prayers live in the ash and the salt of the earth—recognizing our part in the sacred circle, and how everything has a place and purpose in its revolution.

References

Coyhis, D., & Simonelli, R. (2008). The Native American healing experience. *Substance Use & Misuse, 43*:12–13, 1927–1949. doi: 10.1080/10826080802292584

Duran, E. (2006). *Healing the soul wound: Counseling with American Indians and other Native peoples*. Teachers College Press.

Jung, C. G. (2009). *The red book: Liber Novus*, S. Shamdasani (Ed.). W.W. Norton.

Martin, M., & Shaw, R. (2017). How the opioid crisis is affecting Native Americans. Retrieved from https://www.npr.org/templates/transcript/transcript.php?storyId=563551077

Neihardt, J. G. ([1932] 2008). *Black Elk speaks: Being the life story of a holy man of the Oglala Sioux*, the Premiere edition. State University of New York Press.

Takei, M. (2015). A visual picture of the human psyche. *Counseling Today*. Retrieved from https://ct.counseling.org/2015/03/a-visual-picture-of-the-human-psyche/#comment-781546

Tokyo: Kodansha (1983). "Mandala of auspicious beginnings," In *Chibetto "mandara" sh usei* (Tibetan Mandalas: The Ngor Collection). Asian Division, Library of Congress. Courtesy of Kodansha International Ltd., Tokyo (015.00.00) [Digital ID # rb0015]. Retrieved from https://www.loc.gov/exhibits/red-book-of-carl-jung/the-red-book-and-beyond.html

Wiechelt, S. A., Gryczynski, J., & Hawk Lessard, K. (2020). Cultural and historical trauma among Native Americans. In S. Ringel, & J. R. Brandell (Eds.), *Trauma: Contemporary directions in trauma theory, research and practice* (pp. 167–97), 2nd ed. Columbia University Press.

4 My Optional Practical Training Experience

My Perspective as a Japanese Art Therapy Student

Haruka Kawata

One of the most helpful takeaways from my graduate-level class in Social and Cultural Dimensions was to learn that the roots of discrimination come from so-called, othering, and fear of the unfamiliar. People tend to unconsciously attribute differences in opinions to differences in race, ethnicity, and other fundamental unalterable characteristics. Being Asian and an international student is no exception among other targets and contributors in this society of "-isms." However, Asian art therapists are usually overshadowed because there are so few of our stories being told. My narrative demonstrates that racially and ethnically provocative challenges can occur within and against Asian populations, just like any other racial or ethnic minority groups. Sharing more stories of Asian art therapists is a part of "the interplay between making the familiar strange and the strange familiar" (Rosaldo, 1989, p. 39), which is a key to increase the awareness in the field of art therapy. This chapter brings a light into the racial and ethnic challenges a Japanese immigrant faces in the United States, and that could impact the development of a Japanese art therapist's relationships with clients and others. A personal goal I set for myself is to cultivate "mutual empathy," which is "the primary means through which we grow" (Jordan, 2018, p. 29) by telling about my experiences and analyzing it retrospectively. The book *Relational-Cultural Therapy* by Judith V. Jordan was the primary resource that we referenced during our learning in the aforementioned social-cultural class. From this, I learned that just ranting about my experiences would take me nowhere. Ranting would distance me from people with different backgrounds, deprive me of learning about the root of racial, ethnic issues, and power-seeking behaviors. Here, I attempt to break down my stories to recognize my growth as an art therapy student and hope to provide examples of how I learned from these challenges.

Before moving to the United States from Japan when I was 18, I had not been exposed to racially provocative issues because Japan is relatively homogenous in terms of race, ethnicity, and culture. Growing up, there were only a few students and friends with international roots in my neighborhood and schools. Being the majority member had dulled my awareness and sensitivity toward multi-cultural matters, albeit my curiosity toward the world outside had grown. Arriving in the United States opened the door to the unknown, and my interest and ambition fueled my motivation for learning new things. However, I didn't quite understand how systemic discrimination still existed until analyzing it in a graduate school class. I thought everybody was the same who deserved equal rights; to me, racial prejudice was absurd. Innocent and naïve, my lack of awareness was only helping the system of othering, without being sensitive to utilize allyship toward people around me. It was not until I took the class about the social and cultural dimensions that I was exposed to the components and mechanisms of systemic discrimination.

My first challenge happened between a client and me after I completed an undergraduate program and before attending a graduate school. In Missouri, I started working at a local addiction treatment center where I was an intern; later, I became a full-time behavioral health technician. I worked the second shift, from the afternoon hours to the night. One afternoon, one of the clients knocked on an office door and requested that I let her into her room, citing a non-emergency reason. Every client's room was locked all day; the facility policy did not allow clients to return to their rooms for various reasons, including safety. Clients' rooms were all locked, and they were expected to leave their rooms in the morning until the techs unlocked their doors at night. Even though staff members explained the rules during the admission process, many clients continued requesting exceptions. I gently said to the client, I call her Leah to protect her identity, that I was not supposed to unlock the door for her. She begged me and repeatedly said, "Please, Ms. Haruka, please!" I said, "I cannot make an exception only for you unless it is an emergency." I encouraged her to participate in an activity during that time. But we went back and forth several times, and I saw that she was getting angrier, and she was about to explode. Finally, she shouted, "You don't understand! I gotta get into my room RIGHT NOW!" Then she turned around and left the office with fast, inaudible cuss words and the pronounced word "Chinese." Even though I could not hear everything at that moment, the term "Chinese" echoed in my head loud and clear. I called her name and followed her while she rushed down the hallway. Attempting to stop her was of no use. She ignored me and kept going. My feet stopped following her. I knew then I would not be able to talk her down if I was not calm first. Later on, one of my colleagues told me that the client was telling me to go back to a Chinese shop.

I was left in shock. I remember experiencing very confusing emotions and mixed feelings growing in my body. What happened? Shocked ... What? Why? Insulted ...? Embarrassed ...? Confused ... Sad ...? It was one of my first times when I was insulted for being a person of color who was just doing her job. I was at a loss for words and needed to grasp what had just happened. I sighed deeply and sunk in a chair in the middle of the office, replaying the scene in my head again and again. My body still felt stiff. A stream of tears ran on my cheek—Confused, Shocked, Silence. I knew right away that I needed to have a conversation with Leah by the end of the night, if possible (to make an incident report). However, before anything, I needed to think about how to proceed. After a couple of minutes, I was able to push my personal, jumbled feelings aside. Not only did I have to make a report, but I also had to resolve the conflict to build a better professional relationship with Leah so we could continue working together. I told myself that I should leave the office area and work on other tasks. Then, one of the clients who witnessed the incident called my name, quickly handed me a small piece of note, and hastily left. It read: "I don't appreciate what she said to you. You are such a great tech, and you don't deserve it." It made me tear up and reassured me that I was doing the right thing. I finally spoke with Leah, who superficially apologized. However, all I managed to say were how shocked I was and that it wouldn't help her to treat others like that. I didn't know how to approach this matter other than pointing out her wrongdoings. It was not clear to me what was the exact issue, even though I genuinely wanted to help her. Even today, it still feels unresolved. Looking back and after taking the class of social and cultural dimensions, a couple of major things keep bubbling up:

First, why did Leah choose the word "Chinese"? Is calling somebody Chinese supposed to be offensive? Is being Chinese or Asian a negative thing?

Secondly, why did I get offended by being identified as Chinese? Did my cultural pride make me react that way? Or did I have negative associations or antipathy toward Chinese?

And lastly, was that really an act of racism? It felt like racism because Leah attributed to my appearance and identity as an Asian. On the other hand, I'm confused with the remark because it came from a black person, who is also a minority. .

I took the first step by creating art pieces looking back at this incident and how I felt in my body because art often presents something incomprehensible in a visually informative manner. I drew a dark blue meaty heart; the heart represented me during the incident. While I was drawing, I was visualizing a tattoo of a heart with an arrow. I asked myself, "Is the heart pierced? Did it bleed?" Was I "pierced" by the incident? I didn't know. I didn't think it "pierced" me necessarily. Instead, my body perceived it more like pressure from a sharp object. So I decided to draw an arrow jabbing the heart with pinpoint pressure. The color blue felt right for me to express the coldness I felt during the exchange between Leah and me. I put my paintbrush on the desk, looked at this painting, and took a deep breath. Something didn't feel right. Is this how I felt? Was my heart this tender and soft? The arrow didn't convince me either. I felt like I was not honest with my expression. I made a conscious decision to draw an arrow, but did I do so because of the familiar tattoo image? It felt as if I didn't allow myself enough time to explore the right expression of how my body felt during the incident (Figure 4.1).

I grabbed a new sheet of paper. With my eyes closed, I replayed that scene again. My hunch called it right: Something harder and colder—a piece of shattered glass? It felt like it would accurately capture the tension of my physiological environment. I started drawing lines from outside to the center of the paper. As I drew, a swirl of thoughts flew by in the back of my mind about the incident. My heart was not tender and warm ... my heart ... colder and colder ... frozen bloodstream ... nervousness ... being blamed ... being yelled at ... a wall ... defensiveness as a worker ... stretched thin ... no texture and flat ... feeling numb and dull. I then realized that while Leah and I both became stubborn to give in, I was protecting myself with the false security of institutionalized policy, "Because it's a rule." I drew many cracks on the glass, which were

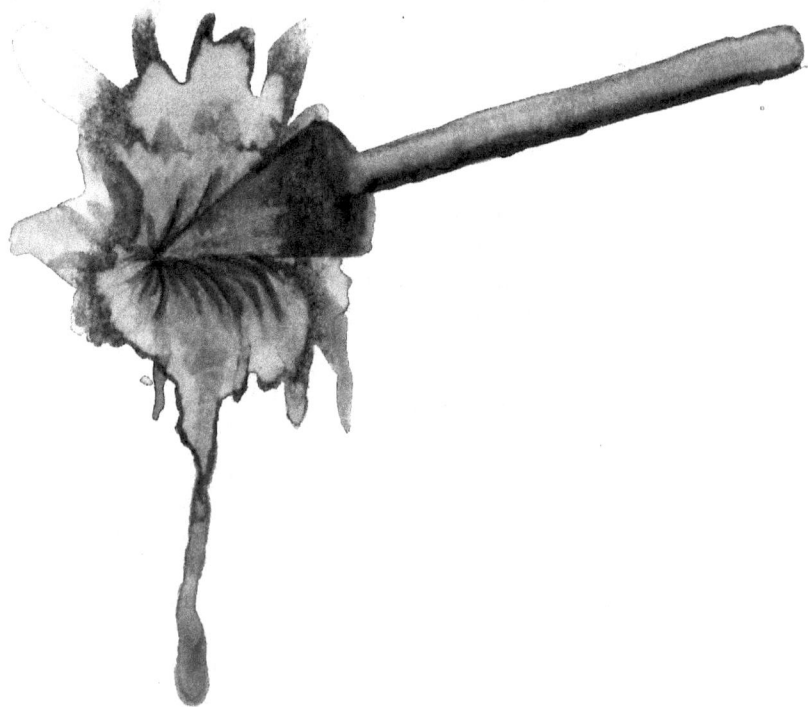

Figure 4.1 Drawing by Haruka Kawata.

the shock and confusion left on my heart. When she snapped at me, my "glass" shattered into pieces. But what exactly cracked my glass? What was the weapon? Was that an arrow or a bullet? I can't see the weapon. As I reflected on the image with a deep sigh, I could see the connection between the lack of weapon and my lack of comprehension about my racial and sociocultural identity. Even though I had intellectually understood them in a classroom, I did not perceive it as my problem because I was someone who was in the majority group in Japan. That let me to emotionally perceive it as a foreign concept until this incident happened (Figure 4.2).

In my experience, there seems to be a stereotypical Asian trope that all Asians are "Chinese." This was off-putting. I gave a thought to why I felt uncomfortable by being identified as "Chinese" after drawing the piece. First, I wanted to be seen as Japanese, not another national identity, and I believe Japan is where I belong. Contrarily, part of me wonders if I was uncomfortable being misidentified specifically Chinese. How would I have felt if I was called Korean or other Asian nationality? I can't help but accept the reality of society that loves labeling. I have been affected by both labeling somebody and myself being labeled by others every day. The research conducted by Pew Research Center showed that 85% of respondents in Japan said that they held unfavorable views toward China, which was the most significant number among all 34 countries participating in this polling (Silver et al., 2019). As disappointing as it is,

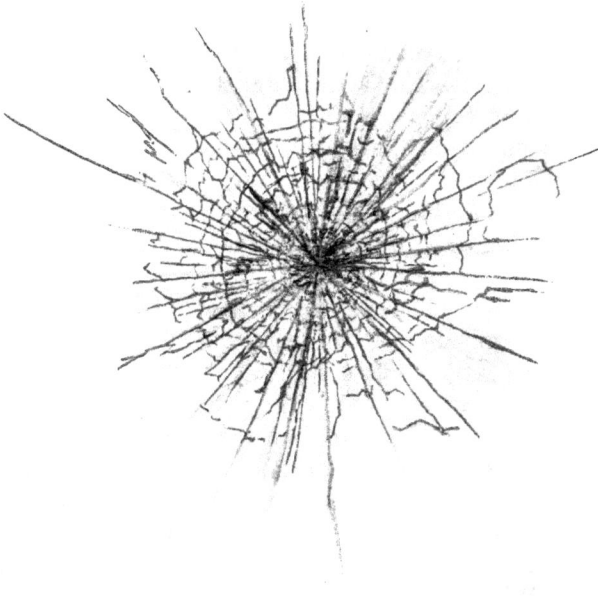

Figure 4.2 Drawing by Haruka Kawata.

it does not surprise me since I know how the Japanese media succeeds, instilling the negative impression of China in Japanese people, including myself, unfortunately. For instance, the Japanese mass media often than not broadcast Chinese tourists' behaviors. Media makes them seem all Chinese people are notorious as talking loud. But talking loud and clear in China is considered a good practice, proving there is nothing to hide, while talking loud in Japan is viewed as a nuisance to people around. Therefore, Chinese tourists enjoying their conversations could be seen rowdy in Japan. Besides, some Japanese media seems to incite anti-Chinese sentiment by emphasizing territorial disputes and controversies surrounding history between Japan and China. History such as Japanese invasion of Manchuria might reinforce our guilt treating Chinese people inhumanely, which also might be disguised as feelings of Japanese antipathy toward China.

On the other hand, I know personally Chinese individuals who have proven favorable to me. My English teacher, who was a Chinese graduate student studying in Japan, was the most delightful and politest person I had ever met. My peer from China in my graduate school is one of my great friends who I can share struggles of being Asian and International. We have supported each other, and it is great to have someone who understands similar cultural and identity struggles. The interactions with them gave me a lovely impression as individuals, in contrast to the depiction of Chinese in the Japanese media. Hays (2001, p. 6) cited, "at the level of the individual, prejudice is lower when one holds the 'knowledge structures' to categorize others as having multiple group memberships" from the researches by Hamilton (1981) and Sun (1993). In my interpretation, this makes persons depicted multi-dimensionally giving them meat and muscles on the flat bone structure and making them real to your imagination. My teacher and my friend are not stick figures that I see on the flat TV screen or smartphone. They are real persons with blood who have different narratives and emotions in their lives. Lumping people all together and labeling is easy, but how much do we know each other individually? Who are we to judge if we don't know different cultures and identities of each other?

Moreover, lumping and categorizing is not only a problem that I need to be careful of applying to other people but also myself. Learning that Japanese people are a "model minority" and "honorary Whites" might have developed my unconscious sense of superiority to other minority group members to some extent. Even though these labels seem to be "positive," it shows the dynamic of sociocultural status from the majority's lens. These labels seem to have an unspoken message, such as "You are still in the minority circle in terms of power. But we grant you some privileges because you follow White people's rules and are productive for the benefits of White Americans." In the same vein, labeling and stereotyping Japanese as "pushover" and "submissive" that sometimes extend to Asians as a group exists. These derogatory terms ravage my dignity because I can't deny the fact I am Japanese, and makes me doubt myself.

Nevertheless, I feel disgust and disapproval of learning about my possible unconscious sense of superiority. This will be very dangerous as a future art therapist. My art revealing my naivety toward racial and ethnic issues causes shame in myself as well because it shows how unconcerned I am of those sensitive circumstances. Being labeled from outside, it causes anger and resistance. It is like a shadow that follows me that I frantically try to escape. My uncomfortable feeling being called Chinese stemmed from being affected by the stream of Japanese media and their conformed notions toward China. As a result, I realize a need to pause myself that allows me to see if my reaction is based on my experience or not, and if not, reeducating myself. The same lesson goes onto my image as Japanese. I don't have control over the Japanese media and people's beliefs from the sketchy information. Still, I do have control over how I can objectively analyze the data and refrain from having conformed ideas and stigmatizing others. While I am exposed to media and stereotypes in my everyday life, I ask myself if the information is real or applicable to my experience. I feel the need to value myself for what I am. With that ability, I can help my future clients see their true value as well.

To explore my question—whether Leah's statement was an act of racism—I turned to the ADDRESSING model, which we learned in our very first semester of graduate school. I hoped to help myself be aware of Leah's background and uncover what beneath the power dynamic between us. This framework allowed me to reflect on my own, and her multi-dimensional identities, with each letter of the acronym, stands for identity categories: Age, developmental and acquired Disability, Religion, Ethnicity, Socioeconomic status, Sexual orientation, Indigenous heritage, Nationality and Gender (Hays, 2001). I had higher power on account of being a behavioral health technician who had a certain control over many of clients' behaviors in the facility, such as reinforcing house rules. Adding to this already complex power dynamic, I was younger, who just recently graduated from a university, a foreigner who was on a working visa, and a person who had never personally experienced substance problems. It might have been humiliating for Leah to be in a locked facility where she was told what to do by me without emotional support from her family and friends. With these views, a few things became clear. First, I didn't know about her personally although I saw her every day until she graduated from the facility. Second, I regained empathy toward her, based on my realization that her life must have been beyond my imagination. I finally accepted that I don't know about her and that it is okay. I don't have to have one simple and clear answer to my question. Further, I experienced empathy toward myself about having my own undefined multi-dimensional identity based on the ADDRESSING model. Learning deeper about Leah and myself made me notice something we share and find similarities, and I hoped that could bring us emotionally closer.

Another trial I have struggled with was with an Asian person. What happens when members of minority groups ridicule each other? There must be a microcosm of oppression among majority and minority because it's about who has "power over" whom, which is "a concept in many societies that people can only feel safe and productive" (Jordan, 2018, p. 136). At a professional conference that I attended as a first-year graduate student, I found myself sitting in one of the support groups. When we discussed the struggles of being minority members, one of the participants, an Asian-American, spoke up. I call her Chloe, who shared that she grew up as an only Asian-American in her small town. I was listening and nodding to her story about the micro-aggression she experienced. It was not long before it took a surprising turn. I was startled when she said that she was offended to be misidentified as an International person.

I froze for a second and said to myself, "Did she really say that? That really hurts me!" I was about to utter comically, but I couldn't. My face probably betrayed my expression, but I repressed my words for the sake of harmony in the support group. Later in that conference, I consulted with one of my peers, who suggested that I talk to Chloe about it. My friend maintained her open body language without dismissing what happened. I knew it was going to be awkward, but my gut also told me to do it right away. When I approached Chloe, my voice was a little bit shaky. I expressed that I was hurt by her words even though I knew her intention was not to hurt anybody in the room. She said she didn't mean to hurt my feelings and quickly apologized, which made me feel relieved on some levels.

In retrospect, Chloe's "International status" statement sounded uninviting because what I heard was "othering" between an Asian-American and a non-citizen. It stung my identity because of my own social ranking as an International student. I'm guessing that she wanted to be perceived as American because she was denied the privilege as a citizen when people from the majority group called her "International." Chloe and I had experienced similar thinking processes and reactions when misidentified for a different ethnicity. I was not pleased to be misidentified as Chinese, as well as the majority called Chloe, an International that upset her. Breaking down the system in which we both exist and understanding our social ranks in society allowed me to see the shared factors between us. We were both exposed to racially challenging remarks, and we struggled to navigate through these experiences in a way that we claim our identity without creating "the other." This drew a sense of patience with Chloe and mutual empathy for both of us.

With the encounter with Leah and Chloe, I am allowed to see the othering and power-seeking behaviors go hand in hand. Leah told me to go back to a China shop showed her intention of othering me from "their group" and excluding me because she did not like my authority as a worker. Likewise, Chloe's statement about not wanting to be grouped with immigrants explained her apprehension about misidentification. I used more empathy than discomfort toward Leah and Chloe to relate because even I'm sometimes not sure which culture I belong to. I can't imagine how hard it has been for Chloe not being treated as an American even though she was born in the United States. Simultaneously, and these incidents displayed that minority group members, including myself, struggle to negotiate our identities. We want to be distinctive but not discriminated against or othered. Another powerful lesson is that we stigmatize and label each other. My conflict with Leah made me realize how much I associated her behaviors with my anxiety around my minority status. However, many of my negative thoughts might not be on her mind. Chloe's stance left me in shock because I first thought she was othering me. I also might have created an unrealistic line between "me/minority" and "them/majority," losing my confidence as a result.

Concluding my narrative, what I have emphasized throughout my chapter is mutual empathy. From the scope of mutual empathy, I need kindness and patience for others and myself as well as toward the exploration of race and ethnicity. To move forward, the key is to forgive each other and ourselves, although maintaining open-mindedness can be hard when my countertransference is active, and there are distorted representations of cultures in mass media. The media and society influence us, and we will continue to be so However, we can still act sensibly upon our decision about racial and ethnic issues and be responsible for it. My goal is to polish my analytical lens during interactions with people to sort out my countertransference, including stigma and labeling, and what they are communicating. This will help me develop myself as a competent counselor and an art therapist. By growing and nourishing our mutual empathy, we will find chances to liberate ourselves from our own mistakes and to move beyond what we believed.

References

Jordan, J. V. (2018). *Relational-cultural therapy* (2nd ed.). American Psychological Association.

Hamilton, D. L. (1981). Stereotyping and intergroup behavior: Some thoughts on the cognitive approach. In D. L. Hamilton (Ed.), *Cognitive processes in stereotyping and intergroup behavior* (pp. 333–353). Lawrence Erlbaum Associates.

Hays, P. A., (2001). *Addressing cultural complexities in practice: A framework for clinicians and counselors.* American Psychological Association.

Rosaldo, R. (1989). *Culture & truth: The remaking of social analysis.* Beacon Press.

Silver, L., Devlin, K., & Huang, C. (2019, December 5). *How people around the world view China.* Pew Research Center. Retrieved January 23, 2020, from https://www.pewresearch.org/global/2019/12/05/attitudes-toward china-2019/

Sun, K. (1993). Two types of prejudice and their causes. *American Psychologist, 48*(11), 1152–1153.

5 An Art Therapist's Perspective on Cultural Humility in Diverse Setting

A Personal Journey from India to the United States of America

Sangeeta Prasad

When I came to George Washington University, the USA, in 1985 to study art therapy, there was no concept of cultural competence or cultural humility. It was through supervision and general course work, as well as several uneasy experiences that I learned to look at my cultural influences. In turn, I saw how these influences affected my therapeutic relationship with my clients and peers and challenged how I translated art therapy teachings from one culture to another. In this chapter, I reflect on my art therapy experiences in India and the United States, my cultural identity, my naive understanding of the various micro and macro cultures, and how supervision helped me understand the influence of culture in therapy. I describe a journey that began before I came to the United States from India to illustrate how developing cultural humility was a part of my learning process. I share my experiences on how different levels of artistic exposure or life experiences of my clients affected my work as an art therapist. Tervalon and Murray-Garcia (1998) stated that cultural humility is to "engage in self-reflection and self-critique as lifelong learners and reflective practitioners" (p. 118). Cultural humility can provide a philosophy for art therapy educators to help students reflect on themselves, understand social power imbalances and help with their lifelong learning (Bodlovic & Jackson, 2018). I will then use the Cultural Humility (HUMBLE) Model to reflect on my experiences. Borkan et al. (2008) described:

H: Be Humble about the assumptions you make about knowing the world from your patients' shoes.
U: Understand how your own background and culture can impact your care of patients.
M: Motivate yourself to learn more about the other person's background, culture, health beliefs, and practices, as well as the unique points of view of their families and communities.
B: Begin to incorporate this knowledge into your care.

L: Lifelong learning.

E: Emphasize respect and negotiate treatment plans. (p. 364)

I grew up in India, a land of diverse languages, cultures, foods, religions, and much more. My grandfather had traveled from Gujarat to Madras, now called Chennai, in search of education and employment. He was one of the first people to leave the community and venture out during pre-independence India. My mom, also from the same community, married my dad, who then left India with my mom in 1955 to study in the United States. My parents returned to India in 1961. I was born in Madras, India, and studied in a Catholic school while I followed Hinduism at home. So my ethnic background is that of a Gujarati who grew up in Chennai, spoke Gujarati, Tamil, Hindi, and English, and studied in a school where there were kids from all over India. This kaleidoscopic background is not unique to me. Everyone has many different subtle as well as overt influences in their life. In my experience, we cannot become "culturally competent," instead, we can be "culturally humble" when we work with people.

My mother had a significant impact on developing my cultural humility. She opposed discriminating against students based on their caste, socioeconomic status, or religion. In her school, she provided an environment where there was an acceptance of differences and celebration of similarities. She grew up in Gujarat, where Gandhi was born, and that influenced her thinking. My mother respected all parents and children who came to her school regardless of their background. Her approach was very different from that of the rest of the schools, where the principal had the power to discriminate and intimidate parents and students. As one of the parents from her school said, "I remember you sitting with my son on the large swing when he was upset, and it is rare to see a principal sit with a child and comfort him."

When I began my art therapy training in 1985, before the Internet and the computer era, my exposure to the United States was through the stories my mom and dad told me about their experiences there. A story I remember my mom telling me was about how cars would come to a halt when she walked down a road since they had not seen a person in a saree (traditional Indian dress). The other major influences were movies and my frequent visits to the US embassy library (air-conditioned and full of books to read). It was in the embassy library that I discovered Edith Kramer's writing on art therapy with children that inspired me to pursue this profession. When I arrived in the United States, I had long black hair, wore mostly Indian clothes, a bindi on my forehead, and a nose ring. I had no experience with the cold or the four seasons. I did not know Thanksgiving and had only celebrated Christmas in school. I was surprised to see professors addressed by their first name, something that I could not dream of doing in India, and people who ate in class, which was a sign of disrespect back home. I found it refreshing that my opinion mattered in class and my assignments. I did not know that most of the learning was from readings, discussions, and writing, unlike the system of teaching back in India, where we listened to lectures and reproduced what we were taught. In my course work and internship, I was encouraged to reflect on my experiences. It began to push the boundaries and preconceived notions about myself, culture, and the connection between human behavior and art. It is what we learn from this process that helps us understand our identity as an art therapist, our experiences with art, and our relationship with our clients.

During the first week of my internship at a special education public school in Washington, DC, my supervisor, a White American, was introducing me to several staff members and students, who were mostly African Americans. I remember wearing a pink salwar kameez (Indian dress), and I had long black hair as well as a red bindi (dot) on my forehead. One young black boy stopped in front of me, looked at me, pointed to the red bindi on my forehead, and asked me if it was a hole in my head, and if the red dot was blood. I was surprised that anyone would mistake a bindi to be a hole in the head. My supervisor asked me in supervision how I felt about this comment, encouraging me to reflect on what I thought maybe going on with the child and what my reactions to this comment were. It allowed me not only to process my response but also to reflect on what impact I was making on the child and how he perceived the world around him. This encounter, and many others to follow, provided me a better understanding of how our perception and experiences affect the therapeutic process and our interactions with each other. Art therapy supervisions became a time where I reflected and became aware of my values and beliefs as well as the children's at the school with whom I worked. One cannot understand the makeup and context of others' lives without being aware and reflective of their background and situation (Tervalon & Murray-Garcia, 1998).

As I began to work with children of ages 7–12 years, I learned a lot about my views and perceptions while understanding the world of these children, which was very different from mine. I began to see how my knowledge of the United States as a rich country because of the wide streets, beautiful buildings, and large cars was changing. I was seeing and learning about the poverty of these families. The children came from broken homes, where they did not get a meal, or there was no one to take care of them. I had witnessed poverty all around me in India, but here I began to see how poverty was hidden from the world and different from what I had seen in India. In supervision, I explored the disparity between the new things I discovered, and I began to understand the history of slavery and colonization in the United States. I explored my feelings about poverty in India and the United States. I learned to be open with the children about their perceptions of their world as well as ideas about my country. Sometimes, the children used cultural differences to connect, and at other times, to alienate or express their anger and sadness. I learned to be curious about our reactions, taking care not to conclude because of a particular cultural bias. Hook et al. (2013) said the following:

> Therapists should not assume that they understand the client's cultural background or experience based on therapists' prior knowledge, experience, or training. Rather, therapists should partner with the client to explore the client's cultural background and experience, in order to determine the aspects of the client's cultural background that may be helping or hurting the client. This attitude of humility may be especially important to the development of a strong working alliance with a client who is culturally different. (p. 361)

I feel that as we begin to work together in any situation, keeping an open mind to understand specific cultural norms helps us broaden our understanding of a given situation. One family we were working with had three children living in a one-bedroom apartment. My supervisor pointed out that this event is not the norm here. I was shocked since in India, a whole family lives in a one-room apartment or house. I expressed my surprise to my supervisor. From my cultural background, the living situation was not a concern, so I did not see any concern about this situation. I had to learn that this culture saw personal space as essential and a right of each person, while in India, we saw the space as belonging to everyone. Understanding the concept of individual versus community space helped me understand how children viewed their relationships.

Another example is about how I non-verbally communicated, "yes" and "no." This is different from the way Americans move their heads up and down to say "yes," and shake their heads left and right to say "no." My supervisor asked me if I could clarify my head gestures. She approached this subject respectfully, stating if it was okay to ask a personal question. She said that she did not understand if I was saying "yes" or "no" since my head moved in a circle. I became aware of how our nonverbal communication can be very different and can lead to misinterpretation. This understanding helps me when I work with people from different cultures. It is vital for the therapist to be aware of her or his cultural background and personal value system and to understand how one's attitudes can interfere with constructive interactions. These understandings are essential prerequisites for becoming a competent art therapist—one who is respectful and considerate of the variations that clients bring to the therapy (Cattaneo, 1994).

Culture affects the way we express ourselves in art. While art is a universal language, it is also influenced by the person's environment, exposure to creative thinking, familiarity with the materials, education level, and other life experiences. How can we, as art therapists, bring in cultural humility into our response to the art in art therapy? On one of my visits to India, I had an experience that opened an understanding of cultural influences on the art of children. I had visited a school that catered to children from lower socioeconomic backgrounds. During the visit, I intended to bring art supplies to the children and have a fun art activity with them. I did not realize that this little visit would begin a lifelong inquiry into the influences of culture on one's art. This experience intrigued me because I became curious about their artwork and the themes they chose to draw. I was able to learn about how they may perceive themselves and their dreams.

During this visit to School A, I asked the children to draw their dream house. I provided the paper and crayons. The children were eager to draw and wanted to use their pencil and eraser; they used the crayons sparingly. They drew detailed pictures of their homes, with kolams (traditional floor drawings in India), temples, flag poles with flags, the interior of their homes, water tankers (a source of water), and many other details of their environment. Their pictures had many features, yet there was not one indication of their dream. The drawings were not what my training in art therapy had taught me about the visual expressions of 10-year-old children. According to Lowenfeld and Brittain (1964), this style of children's drawings is called the "Schematic Stage." Figures 5.1 and 5.2 are artwork collected from this group. I was confused as I had expected to see their dream houses to be something other than what they had drawn. This response led me to collect many drawings of children

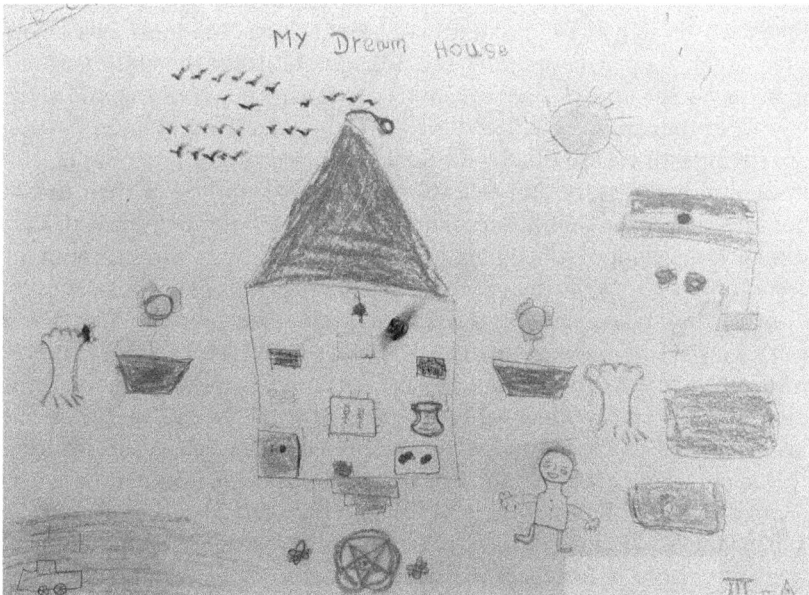

Figure 5.1 Drawing by a child in a school.

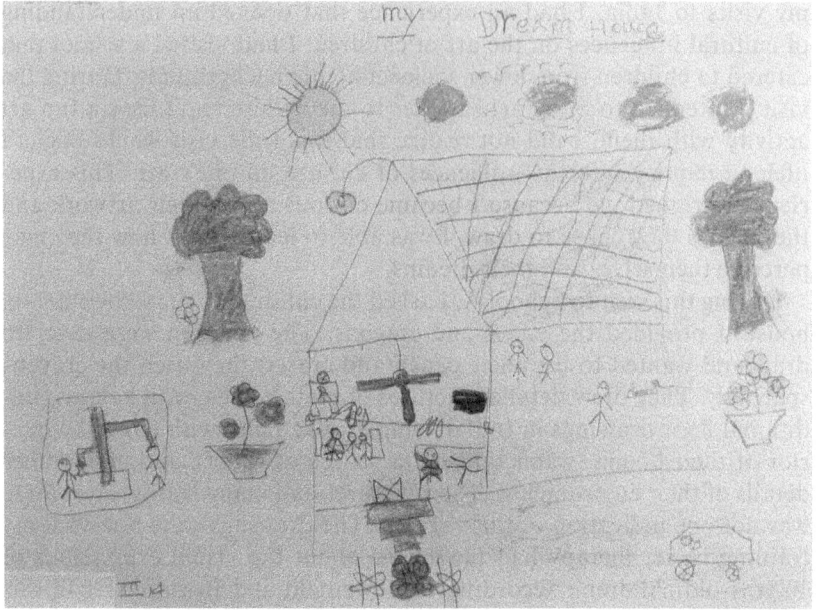

Figure 5.2 Drawing by a child in a school.

from the same age group from various schools, Schools B and C, in the same city and then from other cities (Figures 5.3–5.5). What I found was that even though these children lived less than 20 minutes away from each other, their art was different. I discovered that the children drew many different types of houses, most of which were creative, and some had what they imagined. There were tree houses, flying houses, castles, apartments, or rooms filled with books. Every drawing was unique, creative, and had a story that followed their representation of their dream house. Some of the significant differences were that these children did not have kolams, flagpoles, temples, or water tankers. I was careful about my assumptions about the images from the different groups of kids that were drawn from my art therapy training, as well as my culture. Also, I was wary how these assumptions might impact how I viewed these images while continuing to learn and be curious about these differences in the pictures. The important goal for me was to learn more about what the images meant to the individual and respect the differences and similarities when working with various groups of children. Several art therapists (Campbell, 1999; Doby-Copeland, 2006; Hiscox & Calisch, 2005; Hocoy, 2002; Malchiodi, 2012; Potash et al., 2012) have addressed the implications of culture in art therapy, particularly those of race and ethnicity. However, the influences of socioeconomic background on a child's visual expression remain relatively unexplored in the field of art therapy. Potash

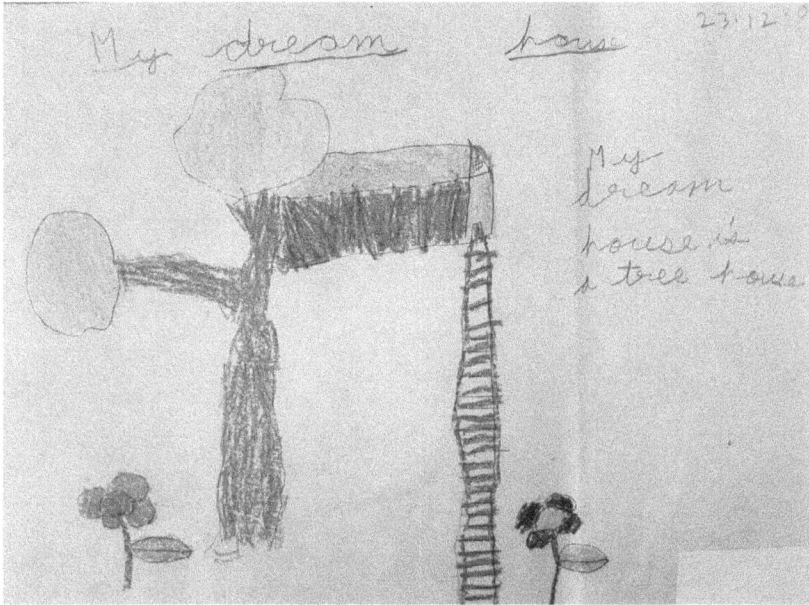

Figure 5.3 Drawing by a child in a school.

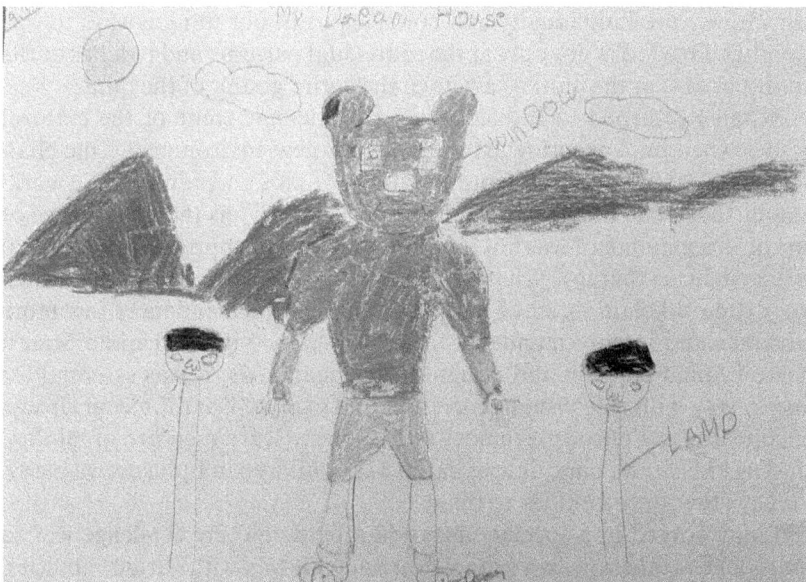

Figure 5.4 Drawing by a child in a school.

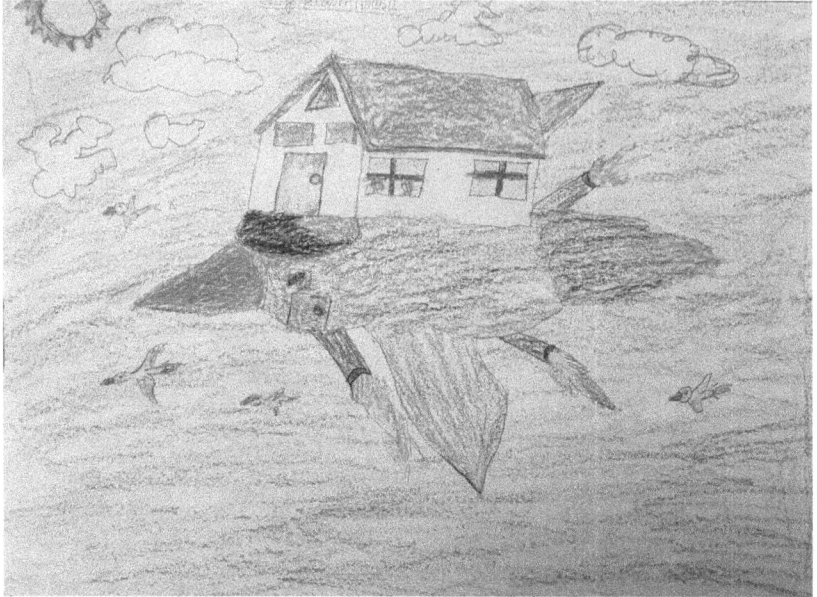

Figure 5.5 Drawing by a child in a school.

et al. (2017) recommend that art therapists be context-sensitive when formulating art therapy instructions and interpreting art. Howie et al. (2013) point out that today's cultural world is like a vast patchwork that makes up who we are individually and connects us in our unique ways to one another. One looks not only at the individual patterns and patches of the quilt but also at the quilt as a whole, the entire gestalt of the quilt.

When I returned to India, I did not anticipate some of the cultural issues when implementing art therapy in a new environment. One challenge I faced in the visual representations of kids and adults while working in India was the use of "Kolam" or "Rangoli" as their first piece of art or in a mandala. I was not familiar with how to approach this cultural art form in art therapy. What were they telling me about themselves when they drew a kolam or made a pretty design in the mandala? I saw more abstract and intense mandalas in my experience in the United States. Here I found colorful and design-centric mandalas. It was essential for me to stay with this visual expression and explore what it meant. It was an opening to a pleasant memory and led me to learn their artistic ability. Just as kids drew comic figures in the west, children in India drew kolams or flags that were familiar to them.

I had worked in a special education school, and my challenge was to introduce art therapy in a school that had children with various abilities. The idea of having individual treatments using art therapy in a school was unusual at that time. To my surprise, parents and teachers were eager to learn about art therapy and how it helps children though I was cautious when introducing the concept. To incorporate art therapy into the current system, building trust with fellow staff members and the administration was a crucial process. We all created a method of working together, creating an art therapy and resource room while we addressed various aspects of the children's emotional, educational, and social needs. When I reflect on how I introduced art therapy within this school setting, I realize I used the HUMBLE model of cultural humility. I was not an expert in starting the art therapy program. Instead, I first became familiar with the existing norms and then incorporated art therapy into the current system with the help of the staff. I had to understand the needs of this community, utilized my knowledge and training of art therapy to meet their requirements. As a result of this experience, I wrote a book, Creative Expressions, Say it With Art, in 2008 for parents and teachers, where I address the importance of art education and the use of art therapy in a school setting.

Working in the United States with fellow Indians and Asians versus working with other nationalities or ethnicities has challenged my understanding of how to work with different groups of people and their view about me. I found that clients who are from India have required a more direct and psycho-educational approach. They also relate to me differently as they feel I understand the language and can communicate their problems otherwise challenging to express in English. It seems like sometimes the client may think that some of the metaphors expressed in the language of origin are lost in translation. Goren (2014) said, "If language is the thread of the therapeutic process, then a foreign-born therapist and a foreign-born patient are weaving together a different kind of fabric, as compared to their native English-speaking counterparts" (para. 5). Goren also points out:

> However, there are potential pitfalls for this dyad. Patient and therapist might be tempted to create a cultural island, thinking in terms of "us" vs. "them," creating what Salman Akhtar, a South Asian born psychoanalyst, calls 'nostalgic collusion' of idealizing the country of origin and together vilifying their new home. They might make assumptions about sameness that blur extraordinary individual experiences and differences. (para. 10)

Now, as I work in private practice with children and adults from various cultural backgrounds, I recognize the critical part of my training is applying multiple art therapy approaches and theories indirectly, preferably with understanding where and with whom I am working. I use mindfulness and cultural humility to understand my clients' presentation of issues and respond with nonjudgmental awareness of my reactions and responses. Together, we unfold the struggles my client is facing, and the art becomes a platform to see, reflect, and learn. I recognize that

I need to be culturally humble at all times. It is a tapestry we are weaving together with care.

References

Akhtar, S. (2004). *Immigration and identity turmoil, treatment, and transformation.* Rowman & Littlefield Publ.

Bodlovic, A., & Jackson, L. (2018). A cultural humility approach to art therapy multicultural pedagogy: Barriers to compassion. *The International Journal of Diversity in Education, 19*(1), 1–9. doi:10.18848/2327-0020/cgp/v19i01/1-9

Borkan, J. M., Culhane-Pera, K. A., & Goldman, R. E. (2008). Towards cultural humility in healthcare for culturally diverse Rhode Island. *Medicine & Health/ Rhode Island, 91*(12), 361–364. http://rimed.org/medhealthri/2008 12/2008-12-361.pdf HYPERLINK

Campbell J., Liebmann M., & Brooks F. (1999). *Art therapy, race and culture.* Jessica Kingsley.

Cattaneo, M. (1994) Addressing culture and values in the training of art therapists. *Art Therapy: Journal of the American Art Therapy Association, 11*(3), 184–186. https://doi.org/10/1080/07421656.1994.10759081

Doby-Copeland. (2006). Things come to me: Reflections from an art therapist of color. *Art Therapy: Journal of the American Art Therapy Association, 23*(2), 81–85. doi:10.1080/07421656.2006.10129646

Goren, D. (2014, June 19). Home away from home: Therapy in a second language when both therapist and patient are immigrants, language assumes special meaning. *Psychology Today.* doi:https://www.psychologytoday.com/us/blog/contemporary-psychoanalysis-in-action/201406/home-away-home-therapy-in-second-language

Hocoy, D. (2002). Cross-cultural issues in art therapy. *Art Therapy: Journal of the American Art Therapy Association, 19*(4), 141–145. doi:10.1080/07421656.2002.10129683

Hiscox, A. R. & Calisch, A. C. (2005). *Tapestry of cultural issues in art therapy.* Jessica Kingsley.

Hook, J. N., Davis, D. E., Owen, J., Worthington, E. L., & Utsey, S. O. (2013). Cultural humility: Measuring openness to culturally diverse clients. *Journal of Counseling Psychology, 60*(3), 353–366. doi:10.1037/a0032595

Howie, P., Prasad, S., & Kristel, J. (2013). *Using art therapy with diverse populations: Crossing cultures and abilities.* Jessica Kingsley.

Kramer, E. (1972). *Art as therapy with children.* Schocken Books.

Lowenfeld, V., & Brittain, W. L. (1964). *Creative and mental growth.* Macmillan.

Malchiodi A. (2012). *Handbook of art therapy.* The Guilford Press.

Potash, J. S., Bardot, H., Moon, C. H., Napoli, M., Lyonsmith, A., & Hamilton, M. (2017). Ethical implications of cross-cultural international art therapy. *The Arts in Psychotherapy, 56*, 74–82. doi:10.1016/j.aip.2017.08.005

Potash, J. S., Kalmanowitz, D. L., & Chan, S. M. (2012). *Art therapy in Asia: To the bone or wrapped in silk.* Jessica Kingsley.

Tervalon, M., & Murray-García, J. (May 1998). Cultural humility versus cultural competence: A critical distinction in defining physician training outcomes in multicultural education. *Journal of Health Care for the Poor and Underserved, 9*(2), 117–125. doi:10.1353/hpu.2010.0233

6   Between Melting Pots

A Filipino American Art Therapist and the Bean Project

Maria Alinea-Bravo

The Philippines, where I was born and raised, is a Southeast Asian country of over 7,000 islands. It has lush mountains and picturesque, breathtaking beaches like those that travel magazines feature. The country is rich in both natural resources and cultural history. Before the sixteenth-century arrival of the Spanish, three major ethnic groups inhabited the islands that are now the Philippines: the indigenous people, Indonesians, and Malays. In 1521 the Portuguese explorer Ferdinand Magellan came to the region and named the island he conquered after his sponsor, King Philip II of Spain. At the time when the Spaniards discovered the area, its regional occupants had many names for the place where they lived. At most, a loose alliance of minor local fiefdoms, the islands, and their inhabitants were without any national identity. While the Spanish found a traditional culture among the people, in the more than 300 years that the Island of Philippines was a Spanish colony, any traditions that the native Filipinos had were effectively supplanted. The people adopted Spanish religion, language, food, and ways of thinking, and thus native cultures were lost. It is said that, if the Spaniards cloistered the Filipinos for 300 years in a convent, the Americans—who bought the islands from Spain after the Spanish-American War—raised the Filipinos in a brothel for 50 years.

In my childhood and teen years, the Spanish and the American were the two dominant cultures that influenced and molded me. The Spanish culture was living in faith, while the American cultural influence that they taught us English, which became the mainstream educational system. Growing up in Manila, the capital city of the Philippines, our family was tight-knit. My grandmother would reinforce the belief that a family that eats and prays together stays together. My elementary and high school days were rigid and firmly structured. When political unrest made continuing my education at home problematic, my family moved to the United States.

While the language was not a problem when I moved, I still had to overcome the culture shock of American lifestyle. Education in the

United States seems to provide students more freedom in a classroom implementing more creative writing exercises and critical thinking processes. But I managed to adopt the change in my educational environment and started college at a large university. But with 80 students in a class, I found myself floundering. Thus, I looked for a small college, and I found one in Connecticut, which my cousin had suggested. Studying while I was away from my family was the most significant challenge and the hardest choice I made. Being on my own, building my sense of self, and making friends with different people—Caucasians, African Americans, and Hispanics—were eye-opening for me who came from a close-knit family and an insular culture. In both my undergraduate and graduate programs, I was one and sometimes the only one of Asian students in my class. However, I consider myself lucky. Albertus Magnus College in Connecticut offered an introduction to art therapy in the Psychology Department. The fusion of art and psychology caught my interest and set me on a path to my current career as an art therapist. It led me to attend a Master's degree program in art therapy at New York University. There I learned better to express myself and to speak up, which helped me develop the most definite sense of self. Being among a minority in my classes, I did not feel less of who I was or less than anyone else. Instead, I thoroughly enjoyed the independence living on the East Coast.

While I was a graduate student, I worked part-time at Metropolitan Hospital in NYC. Many other students worked there part-time, and I was surrounded by my coworkers, who came from different ethnic backgrounds. The combination of going to school and work was burdensome. As a student, I had ample time to do other things. But studying and working at the same time left me with only one free day a week. Once I received my Master's degree, I worked my way up from a provisional part-time worker to a full-time civil servant employee for the city.

Currently, I am the only Asian art therapist in my current department at Coler Rehabilitation and Nursing Care Center in Manhattan. It is a long-term facility for residents with medical conditions that leave them unable to take care of themselves without any place to live. Our residents range in age from 30 to 100 years old with diagnoses such as chronic heart failure, hemiplegia from gunshot wounds, multiple sclerosis, traumatic brain injury and Alzheimer's disease and other forms of dementia. Both our residents and staff are mostly New Yorkers who hailed from different countries and thus have varied backgrounds. In addition, their homes of origin range from the Philippines, Haiti, the Dominican Republic, several African countries, Jamaica, Trinidad, India, and the United States.

That unique situation results in some arresting moments. It is interesting to see how residents and staff comment on my physical features.

I am a typical Filipina with brown skin, which means that I am often mistaken for someone who comes from a foreign country. "Where are you from?" they often ask. While most staff guess I am Filipina, some residents assume that I am Chinese, Mexican, or even from the Caribbean islands. When I explain that I am Filipina, the next question is usually, "Are you a nurse?" That is not a surprising assumption, as the Philippines might a good resource for nurses to work around the world. When I respond that I am a therapist, many assume that I am a physical or occupational therapist. The word therapist is most often not associated with art. Being the only Asian and an art therapist can be isolating. To overcome the isolation, I reach out to colleagues outside work and have a peer support group once a month. I am thankful for the fellowship that I have found in the group. Also, the annual art therapy conference, where they allow me to be part of the community, refreshes, energizes, and renews my mind and spirit. They make me feel better at what I do and give me a purpose and a validation as an art therapist.

When I talk with my coworkers and the residents, I use my Filipino features and cultural background to my advantage to connect with them to learn where they come from. It leads to a discussion about how their lives were in their home countries, including talking about food. In many places, I've discovered, beans are a common element in local diets, so we find commonality there, as beans play an important role in Filipino cuisine as well. This discovery helped lead me to one of my most successful projects—the Bean Project, mixing food with art. For me, the beans represent my early childhood. Many of our meals use a variety of beans like mung and string beans. My residents and I shared cultural experiences in the lowly legume, which gives me a safe starting point to work with culturally diverse residents. I use art to foster residents' minds and spirits just as beans have nourished their bodies and physical well-being. My ethnicity, identity, and role as an Asian art therapist all played essential parts in the Bean Project, which I am about to explain. All connected for me, and they are just as much a part of my residents' lives as well. So I used beans to educate residents and staff about what art therapy is.

The germ of the idea for the Bean Project came from a course I took during the 2018 American Art Therapy Association conference. The Bean Project was a simple and straightforward one that I thought was adaptable to the needs of my residents. I brought it back to my workplace as part of our Art Exhibit 2019. Turning beans into art forms helped me to focus on the diversity of cultural backgrounds in the facility. The art therapy groups I conducted had four or five participants each—African Americans, Caribbean Islanders, and Asians. They were roughly 50–83 years old. Here is a description of the project.

Materials: "10×10" pieces of cardboard with a circle drawn in the center; some simple glue; and beans of various colors, white, black, red, and pink. I included corn kernels and sunflower and pumpkin seeds as well, though they are not essential.

Method: I introduced the beans as a jumping-off point for discussion, identifying each grain or seed, touching them, and even tasting them.

This stimulated not only the residents' various senses but also their memories, as we discussed the beans as part of each resident's culture and how each bean can be cooked. A Jamaican resident, for example, mentioned cooking them as a soup; a woman from Grenada added beans in her stew, and a woman born and raised in New York expressed a fondness for corn to make popcorn and to eat sunflower and pumpkin seeds as snacks. An African-American resident said, "Beans are nourishment," and they all reminisced, linking the past to the present that "helped seniors identify and recognize their strengths, talents, and uniqueness" (Buchhalter, 2011, p. 286). Sharing stories about bean recipes, myself included, encouraged us to open up by discussing how we ate growing up.

A shared family meal brought out the importance of connecting to love ones and how important togetherness is, as the residents became a temporary family making art together. I then gave each participant one of the cardboards. I directed them to start with one bean in the middle, then go outward to fill in the circle. Some independent participants just followed the instructions and started the project on their own while I went around each resident to see whether they needed assistance. I helped some participants with impaired motor skills squeezing the glue bottle. Malchiodi (2010) remarked, "Sometimes, an art therapist literally becomes the hands for an individual; an adult with a debilitating medical illness may need me to cut and arrange photos for a collage" (para. 5). The participants decided individually what beans they used and what design they put on their board. As they completed their work, everyone shared their artworks, and everyone admired and praised each one. We put all the finished works together as a whole, which made an effort into a collective art piece.

The participants benefitted from the Bean Project in the following ways: It helped the residents to focus on the project to enhance their attention span, the project gave them a purpose to enjoy the creative process, and reminiscing about the beans increased their self-esteem and improved their socialization. Figures 6.1–6.4 feature some of the residents' artworks.

I presented this Bean Project during our facility's annual art exhibit. It was well received and helped educate the rest of the staff about the

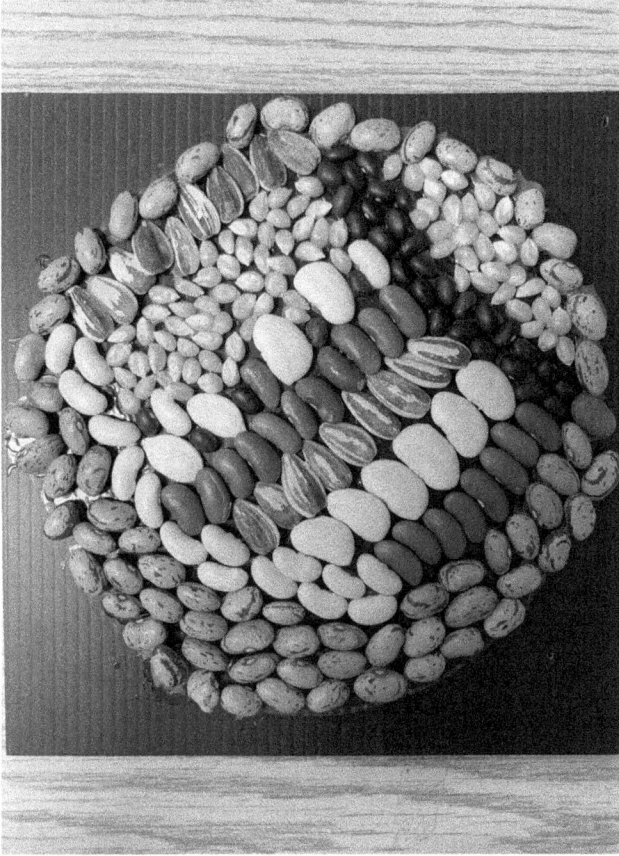

Figure 6.1 Art project by a resident in a nursing home, NYC.

creative process of art therapy. Staff members were impressed at how I came up with a simple project that has a clinical component and therapeutic value. Their feedback ratified how what I do as an art therapist is different from other disciplines.

The Bean Project came about as I looked closely at the residents living in the nursing care center. Integration of cultural diversity is a vital part of the workplace as residents and staff, who came from so many different ethnic backgrounds, and there are unique stories to share. The Bean Project, therefore, celebrated our ethnicity and safely transformed itself into art. It bound us together and became a thread to acknowledge our differences empathically.

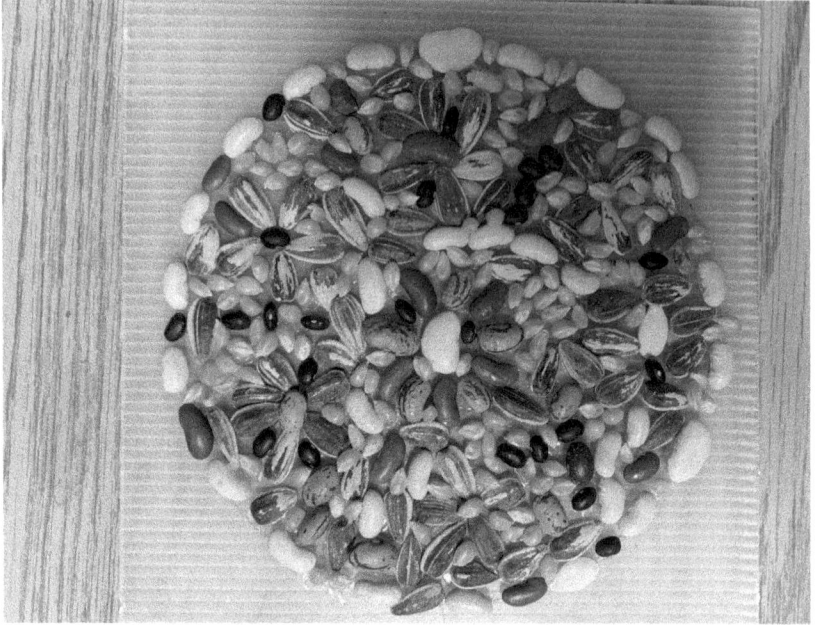

Figure 6.2 Art project by a resident in a nursing home, NYC.

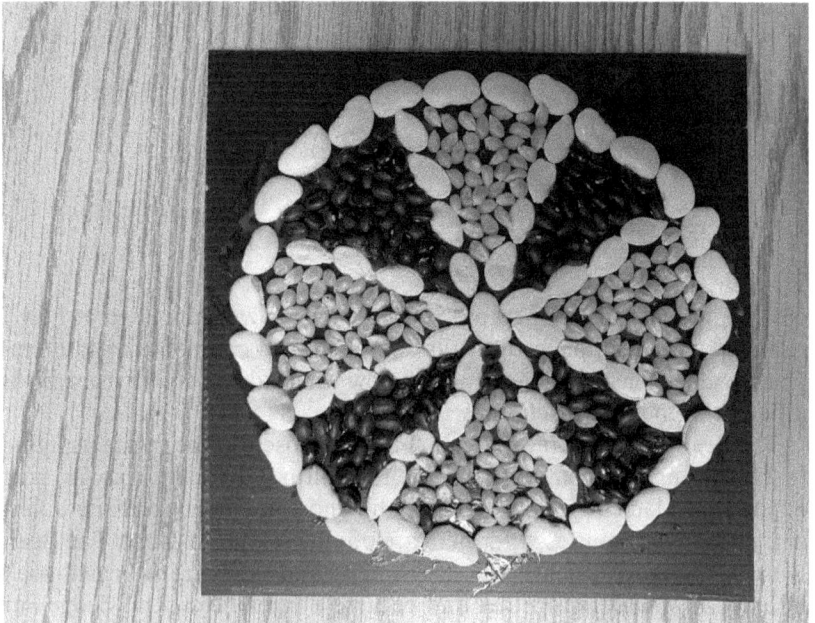

Figure 6.3 Art project by a resident in a nursing home, NYC.

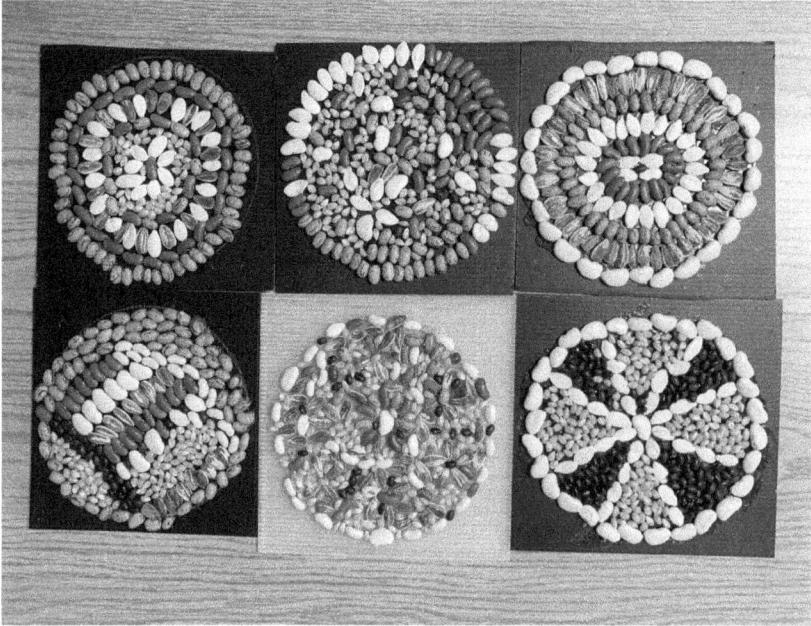

Figure 6.4 Combined works by the participants.

References

Buchalter, S. (2011). *Art therapy and creative coping techniques for older adults.* Jessica Kingsley Publisher.

Malchiodi, C. (October 31, 2010). *Cool art therapy intervention #1: The art therapist's third hand.* Psychology Today. Retrieved from https://www.psychologytoday.com/us/blog/arts-health/201010/cool-art-therapy-intervention-1-the-art-therapist-s-third-hand.

7 Unrealistic Expectations and Harsh Realities

Navigating Career Development as an Asian Art Therapist

Ashley Severson

I grew up as a second-generation Filipino American immigrant in New Jersey in the 1990s. In 1970, my dad was about two years old when he moved to Liverpool, NY because his dad had a job opportunity as a chemical engineer, while my mom came to America in 1990 when she was 27 years old. My parents met in the United States and married in 1992. The next year, I was born, making me the eldest daughter and first grand-daughter. My two sisters followed in 1996 and in 2000. For most of my childhood, we lived in a wealthy, predominantly White suburban neighborhood in southern New Jersey. Growing up in America, I did not have a deep tie to my Filipino heritage. My mom had a richer cultural link than my dad, possibly because she lived in the Philippines throughout her childhood and her young adulthood. She spoke fluently in Tagalog and cooked plenty of Filipino dishes. In contrast, my dad did neither. My upbringing is more similar to my dad's, in which I assimilated to American culture and lost touch with my Filipino heritage. My experience may not be generalizable to all Filipino Americans, but this is my story growing up in a New Jersey household, being a child of immigrants, and the oldest sibling.

Growing up, I learned some aspects of Filipino culture from going to family gatherings, listening to the language, sharing Filipino dishes, calling my aunts and uncles, "tita" and "tito," and asking for blessings from older relatives which meant taking the elder's hand and placing it on your forehead as a sign of respect. The hobby that separated myself from the rest of my family was my desire to create art. As a child, my escape was through isolation, journaling, and creating art in my bedroom. I enjoyed making art, and it gave me a sense of control, confidence, and passion. I would post my anime artwork all around my room with an abundance of color, not noticing that it was my safe space using just colored pencils, markers, tape, and computer paper (Figure 7.1). Family members seemed drawn to my artwork. Some asked if I would sell my drawings or be an artist. At the time, I did not see myself as someone who would sell my art since I enjoyed the art process and the emotional attachment to the art.

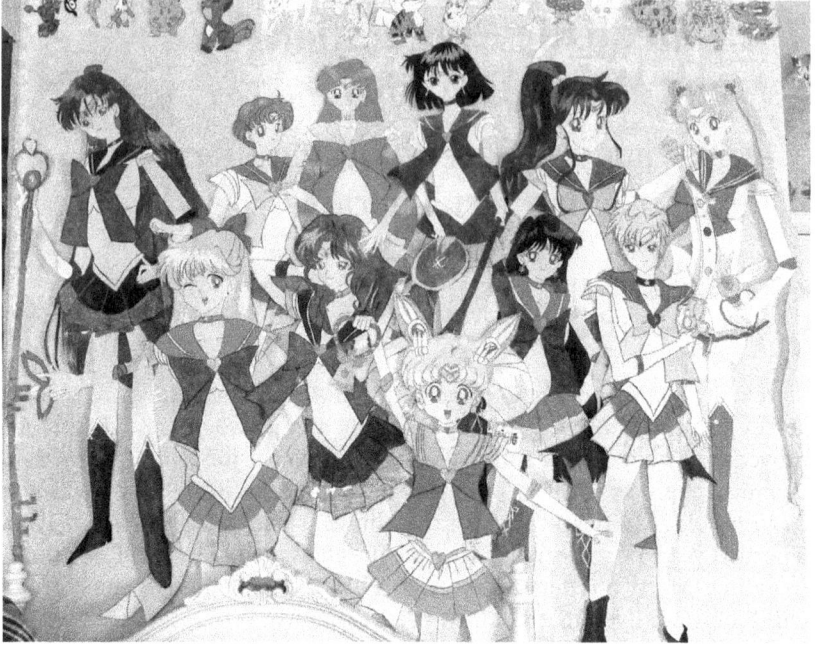

Figure 7.1 Drawing by Ashley Severson.

As much as I recall having such a playful childhood, there were events that people did not see behind closed doors. My family had high expectations for me. I felt pressured to succeed in their eyes so I could not disappoint them. Whenever I would do something wrong in my dad's eyes, I would be humiliated and physically punished by him. Whenever I would do something wrong in my mom's eyes, I would be shamed and emotionally demeaned.

My mom, who was a first-generation immigrant, felt that it was everyone's dream to see the United States. She was the second youngest of her nine siblings, who grew up in Manila, Philippines. Her dad was a businessman and provided for the family while her mom was a stay-at-home parent. Through her dad, she saw having a successful career could provide for the family is viewed as "perfect," while someone who can take care of the family is viewed as "prosperous." Her siblings were raised to become businessmen, bankers, and doctors. Her professional goals were to practice pediatric medicine, study for her boards, and complete her residency. After she and her sister received their US visas, which were difficult to obtain, they moved to the United States in 1990. Throughout her first year in the United States, she felt homesick because she missed her family and the warmer weather. She accomplished her professional goals while working a full-time position.

In contrast, my upbringing was different from my mom's in various ways. The culture was surprisingly not seen as prioritized. When my sisters and I were born, she wanted to make sure we were set up for successful career as if it was the only "checkbox" she cared. I was lucky enough to live in an affluent neighborhood and attended a well-regarded public high school, which helped me with my education. As long as I can remember, my family envisioned me going to medical school because I would have a high paying position as a doctor and follow my mom's footsteps as a pediatrician. As a child, I told my relatives, "I am going to be a dentist or a doctor." My relatives praised that and validated me, but as I grew older, I did not see myself in those roles anymore.

Sometimes, people can think of a profession as a child, but others might question that as teens or throughout their lifetime, "Who do I want to be? How do I want to spend the rest of my life?" As a young adult, I declared my path to becoming an art therapist. Though, I endured many obstacles before the start of my art therapy journey. Family expectations and socio-economic status strongly influenced those challenges. My career identity started to take form in high school. I began to look into my strengths, interests, and values. I knew I had a passion for helping others, but I was unsure how I wanted to pursue that. In high school, I took AP Psychology, where I acquired an interest in learning about mental health and behavior. My family told me I was supposed to know what field to pursue while I submitted my college applications though I still had no idea. I felt alone and anxious during this process. I felt surrounded by family members, telling me what I should do as if I was going to be this perfect person in their eyes. I decided to take up Psychology as a major since I gained an interest and curiosity in that field.

When I began college, I knew that I wanted to move out of my household and start a fresh chapter in my life. I decided to attend Drexel University in Philadelphia, Pennsylvania. I loved the transition from living in a suburban environment to a diverse city. The 25 minute drive from home gave me enough distance to be independent but still keep in touch with family. Being away from what I saw as a harsh environment, I experienced growth in infinite ways. I met peers who also did not know what to pursue, which made me feel validated. I finally felt accepted by my peers, which allowed me to discover who I wanted to be personally and professionally. Drexel University enabled me to work at various internship sites that allowed me to explore the mental health field and branch out to numerous opportunities.

I was 20 years old when I interned with the Ronald McDonald House Family Rooms at the Children's Hospital of Philadelphia, where I met families on the oncology and cardiac floors. I welcomed people into the McDonald's Family Rooms that consisted of living rooms, kitchens, and laundry rooms. This position allowed me to actively listen to caregivers as they processed their child's progress and their time in the hospital.

Those experiences shaped me to become who I am today as someone who wants to make a positive impact and build relationships with others. On certain days, an Asian American art therapist worked with caregivers in the kitchen area. It was a fantastic opportunity for me to meet an Asian American art therapist and ask about the profession. She mentioned that she received her art therapy graduate degree from Drexel University, so I looked into the program and the profession. About a few months later, I attended Drexel's Art Therapy open house, observed a class, and met art therapy students. I decided to minor in fine arts and psychiatric rehabilitation, which was a crucial step to officially deciding to pursue art therapy.

I was very excited to share with my family that I wanted to pursue art therapy but very nervous at the same time. My family and relatives had no idea what art therapy was and expressed reservations about my decision. My mom, in particular, was not supportive of me becoming an art therapist. She was the leading family member who wanted to pave and choose my profession. She told me, "You won't be successful if you decide to be an art therapist," and that was tough to hear. It's funny that my family supported the idea of me being an artist earlier in my life but had difficulty understanding my role as an art therapist. From my experience, it seemed that my family did not prioritize mental health compared to physical health. If I did not feel well or sick, my family, my mom, in particular, focused on physical ailments and pain but not the mental health aspects. I would be called "sensitive" for showing or sharing my feelings, so they were hardly shared moving forward. From my experience in a Filipino family, emotions such as sadness or fear were rarely expressed or looked down. If I showed those emotions in public, I would feel humiliated or uncomfortable. Because of how my dad physically punished me and my mom's harsh statements, I rarely shared those hurtful experiences with anyone growing up. When someone asked me about those experiences, I played it off, saying, "I'm okay," but of course, I was still hurting. Asking for help made me feel like I was incapable of taking care of myself.

Even though my mom disapproved of my decision, I did not want to give up something that could be my passion. I know that I took control of my career path in undergrad, but it finally started to take off when I applied for art therapy graduate school. I decided to attend George Washington University's Art Therapy Program in Alexandria, Virginia. Attending classes and going to personal therapy allowed me to process my experiences and gain a deeper understanding of myself. I focused on my family heritage and upbringing. At the same time, I took Social and Cultural Diversity, Art Therapy with Adolescents, Marital & Family Art Therapy Counseling, and Art Psychotherapy & Trauma II. I did not realize there were many aspects from my upbringing that were buried deep, just waiting to resurface. I gained insight into the formation of my identity and how it led me to the art therapy field. From someone who had challenging childhood experiences, I can understand how time in therapy can be intense but essential in self-growth.

My first class in Social and Cultural Diversity allowed me to explore my teenage years using markers and chalk pastels. I decided to focus on my struggle with being a Filipino American. In high school, I felt out of place from my Filipino American classmates. At times, they ridiculed me and told me, "You are not Asian enough, you are White," as if I was not good enough because I was sometimes unfamiliar with certain Filipino traditions. Though some joked about this concept, it never sat well with me. I still struggle today with my cultural identity after being shamed for not being "good enough." Therefore, I tend to disconnect away from possibly shaming because I become easily triggered by microaggressions and expectations. I created a self-portrait that represented "the between" of being American and Filipino (Figure 7.2). My artwork expresses my struggle to meet and deal with people's cultural expectations, especially as an adolescent/young adult. There is an apparent split in my portrait. The arrows and red marks represent the harsh comments I dealt with. The zipper represents how I am afraid to communicate feeling hurt and

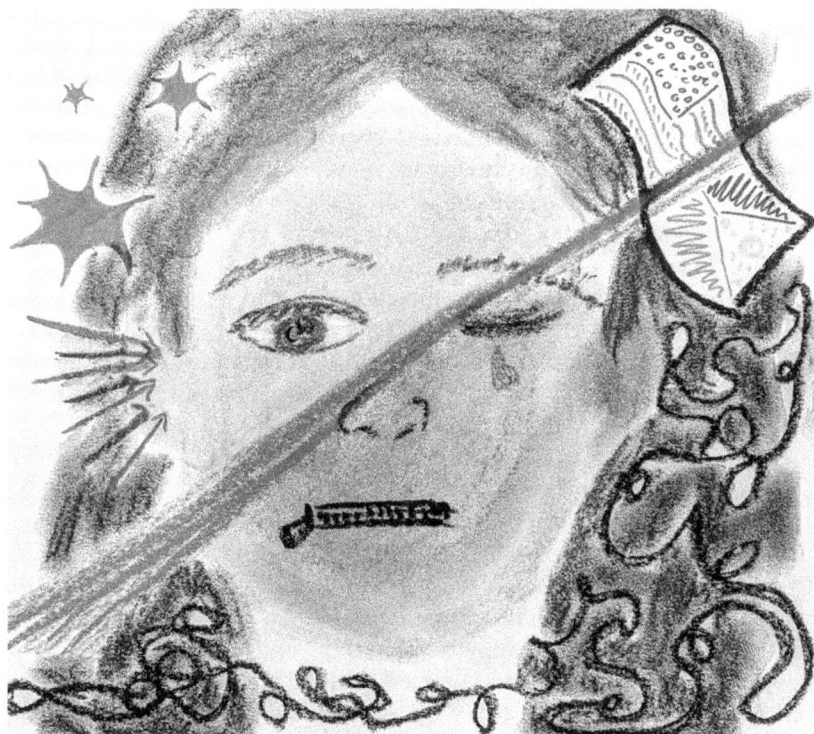

Figure 7.2 Drawing by Ashley Severson.

shamed. The curvy black lines symbolize my confusion and the entangle-ment of, "Well, who am I supposed to be?" It feels unfair to neglect my heritage as a Filipina, so it is a life-long process that I am still working on to embrace it.

During my time in the program, it was known that there was a need for broader racial and cultural representation in the art therapy field. I received emotional support from my professors, but I seemed to be missing a racial/ethnical component. I wanted to hear and connect with people of color. I served as co-chair of the Multicultural Committee, and a group of students created an art therapist of the color group. We only met a few times after we established this group. There was never enough time to discuss how being a minority affected us in the field since we had such busy schedules though it was necessary to have a safe space to talk about diversity issues. Then one day, my partner and I decided to visit my family in Maui for a winter break. My uncle on Oahu works for Hawaiian Airlines so that we could use standby for a lower price. Little did we know, this trip would be a turning point in our careers and lives.

We enjoyed our time there. People told us that our professions, me as an art therapist and my partner as an attorney, were much needed on the island. My partner and I did not talk about the possibility of moving to Maui until he had a job opportunity during my final year in gradu-ate school. I was hesitant about the idea of starting my career in Hawaii when there was no art therapy licensure on the islands, so I felt unsure if I could practice as an art therapist. I knew I wanted to at least work in a state that recognizes the profession. With having this one shot at mov-ing to Hawaii, I decided not to pass up this opportunity. But I received support and suggestions from my professors in graduate school. I used the Art Therapist Locator on the American Art Therapy Association website to connect with art therapy graduates who were either native or new to the island. At the time, there were none on Maui, which was my potential moving location. Most art therapy graduates were on Oahu or the Big Island. I connected with them and gained an understanding of how to begin my art therapy career in Hawaii.

Once my partner and I made this moving decision together, I began to reach out to mental health organizations to create a foothold before our move in August 2019. In December 2018, I made a connection with a non-profit called Maui Youth and Family Services. It was an opportunity to work with teens battling substance abuse issues. I shared that I would move there in August, but if they could keep my application once I moved to the island, I would be happy to discuss the opportunity. It is amazing how things turned out because once I finally moved to the island; they reached out to me about setting up an interview. During my interview, my interviewer seemed amazed at how my art therapy experience has helped my previous clients, and she was open to allowing teens to use art therapy. I was proud of myself for finding a position that gave me the flexibility and opportunity to practice as a counselor using both talk and art therapy. Though I previously worked with adults with substance abuse, I wondered what challenges awaited me working with teenagers with substance abuse issues and settling in Maui.

First, it was vital for me to learn about the history of the island. Maui is called the "Valley Isle" and is the third-largest island in Hawaii (Polancy, 1999). Maui county includes three other smaller islands: Molokai, Lanai, and Kahoʻolawe. The vibe is very laid back compared to living in Philadelphia for six years and by Washington D.C. for two years. According to the U.S. Census Bureau (2019), 167,417 people live in Maui County. Maui has various settings: rural areas, beaches, the valley, mountains, and luscious green farms, stretches of vacation homes and hotels, and touristy towns. Many locals have seen how commercialized and city-like Oahu has become that they do not want to see their island follow the same path.

On Maui, sugar plantations were abundant and stretched across 36,000 acres (Sugar Museum, 2018). The sugar cane plantations began in Maui around 1848, so this introduced new jobs for the people of Hawaii and immigrants from China, Japan, Korea, Portugal, Puerto Rico, and the Philippines. Since the immigrants spoke different languages, communication was difficult. For them to communicate, they came together and formed "pidgin," which was mainly influenced by Tagalog, Hawaiian, Japanese, Cantonese, and Portuguese speakers (2018). When I started working on Maui, I heard pidgin phrases that I was not familiar with, which became a language barrier for me. It seems that my clients and co-workers used pidgin when they shared their stories. When I asked some kids what their phrases meant, some would respond and explain, but others reacted because I did not comprehend. It would not be right of me to ignore the fact that I did not know the meaning of their statements, but now I understand it more clearly. Common phrases such as "Grinds," means to eat and, "Talk Story," means to chat or gossip. "Da kine" is used when you cannot find a simple explanation of action or word when it does not come to mind. For example, "What was the name of that movie, ya know da kine."

Though Hawaii is a US state, Hawaii has a unique blend of cultures and backgrounds that makes it very different from other States. According to the Research Economic Analysis Division (2018), the following percentages of people living in Hawaii self-identifying alone or part as Asian is 57.2%, White is 43.4%, Native Hawaiian and other Pacific Islander is 26.9%, Black or African American is 3.6% and, American Indian and Alaska Native is 2.7%. There is no majority population on Maui, which is what makes it so unique. Even though there is no majority group does not mean all groups on the island experience life in the same way. Hawaii was first ruled by those of Polynesian descent then by foreign wealth. Looking back at Hawaii's history, Hawaii was overthrown and taken over by the United States. At first, White newcomers wanted to bring innovations and industry, which were welcomed mainly by Hawaiian royalty. Over time these wealthy influential White individuals accumulated power and status among the Hawaiian elite, which allowed for the eventual overthrow of the government, imprisonment of Queen Lili'uokalani, and status as a US territory (Polancy, 1999).

At work, I noticed a client call my White client, "haole." I was not sure if it was derogatory or its true meaning behind it. I learned that the term originated when the first Caucasians arrived on the islands. Then I became aware of Hawaii's history as to why the power dynamic exists among Native Hawaiians and Caucasians. When calling someone "haole," there is no weight behind it compared to a White person using derogatory language towards a minority. Despite the real differences between the language and its impact, I felt some sense of empathy for my White client. I felt that my client was shunned away for being White, which brought back memories when I was shunned away for not being "Filipino enough." When the clients hung out together outside, I noticed that my White client asked if he could create art together instead. One of my reasons for pursuing art therapy was to give people a safe place to express themselves, and this was an opportunity.

Given the cultural expectations from my family, I wondered if my move to Hawaii, a place with a prevalent population of Filipinos, would place new expectations on me. That moment brought me back to a time in graduate school when I viewed my cultural identity when I drew my identity as a Filipino American and the criticism I received for having a different cultural upbringing. From that experience, I saw how being different made me feel unaccepted. I think that I am struggling with two fronts of my identity, (1) living in Maui where I look "local" and (2) being in between being American and Filipino. Because of my skin tone, many "locals," thought I was from the islands. From surrounding myself with those who grew up on the island, they have pride being "local." There seem to be various definitions or criteria to call yourself a local. I have heard, "You need to be born on the island," "You accept and do not change anything about the island," "You are part of the community," and "They commonly speak pidgin." I was told that "I am a local" or "I am not a true local," so there is confusion as if I am placed in one or the other.

When it comes to self-disclosure, I think about why I disclose and if that benefits the client or me. I do not share with my clients that I am from the mainland because I am afraid that I will be treated differently for being "from the mainland" and not from Hawaii. In the past, I felt shunned from groups for being different, so I noticed that I protect myself from that. When I do share that I am from New Jersey, I tend to quickly show a connection with Maui by saying I have a family that has lived on the island for 20+ years. It brings me comfort, selfishly trying to validate to be treated the same as a typical local.

My art therapy journey has just begun. I am in the process of establishing my place here on the island personally and professionally. My chapter gave me much insight into my upbringing and finding my place in this world. There is an abundance of opportunities to learn from Hawaii's mix of cultures, and it has been a refreshing experience working with a multi-diverse population. There is a strong need to have more art therapists of color in the field, and I see the need, especially here in Hawaii. I think it is important to hear more from those in Hawaii as practicing art therapists. I hope that my story gives you a unique perspective of a second-generation immigrant trying to navigate her way towards a creative career path. I patiently teach my family about art therapy and the benefits of supporting others through the art process as I work with teens, who are unfamiliar with the profession. It is my mission to educate more about art therapy, so their idea of therapy can feel more welcoming and diminish the stigma behind the treatment.

References

Polancy, T. (1999). Politics and issues. *So you want to live in Hawaii: A guide to settling and succeeding in the islands* (pp. 37–50). Barefoot Publishing.

Research Economic Analysis Division. (2018). *Hawaii Population Characteristics 2018*. Retrieved from http://files.hawaii.gov/dbedt/census/popestimate/2018_county_char_hi_file/Pop_char_hi_2018_final.pdf.

Sugar Museum. (2018). *Explore Maui's sugar history*. Retrieved from https://sugarmuseum.com/.

United States Census Bureau. (2019). *Quick facts Maui County*, Hawaii. Retrieved from https://www.census.gov/quickfacts/mauicountyhawaii.

8 Find Lost Name

Self-Reflection on the Journey of Being an Art Therapist

Chia-Ling Kao

Chia-Ling Kao Is My Name

In 2001, a Japanese animation, "Spirited Away," written by Hayao Miyazaki, portrays a spirit world that transforms people's identities into slaves unconsciously. Throughout the movie, the audience learns the secret of finding one's way home is to recognize one's name. The film metaphorically spoke of my experience as a foreigner in the United States. I was lost for years as a spirit while I pursued my career in art therapy.

Throughout my career in America, I have been called, "Chia," "Chio," "Chili," "Chocola," "Jia," "Chian," etc. paired with various pronunciations. The hyphen in my name connects two words, which combine as one given name, although most people assume that the "Ling" is my middle name. Some people who could not remember my name called me, "Lucy Liu." For me, it was still better to be called "that Chinese lady" at work. In the medical setting, many Asian professionals work as physical therapists and occupational therapists, but not many worked as creative arts therapists. For a time, I felt that it was my responsibility to teach native English speakers the beauty of Traditional Chinese characters, which are created with metaphors and arts. I have always enjoyed educating my colleagues about my culture and explaining the differences between Chinese and Taiwanese or Taiwan and Thailand. Still, in the end, I gave myself an accessible name, "Jamie" to fit into social circles. My heart desired to establish an identity associated with ambition, articulation, or astuteness in New York.

In time, life was uncomplicated for me if I went by the name, "Jamie." For job hunting, using an easy-to-remember Western name on my résumé would boost my chances of being selected. During the last semester of my graduate program, to secure employment, I would wake up at 6:00 in the morning and send out at least 20 résumés every day to various places. Since more recreational positions were available than specialized art therapist positions, I made a point to outreach all of the nursing homes in the United States, as they were more likely to have art therapy programs. Because of the positive experience of studying creative arts therapy in school, I went after the opportunity to stay in the United States to equip myself with more art therapy skills. Becoming a board-certified or state-licensed art therapist was a significant recognition of my profession, whether or not I decided to return to Taiwan.

Despite my aspiration for establishing myself in the art therapy profession, my anxiety hit the roof when I found myself unable to attain a position for six months after graduation. Most international students who desire to stay in the United States face the issues of applying for a work visa with limited time and low chances. On top of those challenges, the individuals' college majors also limit opportunities. When I was just on the brink of giving up, an alumna of my school referred me to her workplace for a part-time art therapist position. I then started working two hours a week with the geriatric population. I was proud that I had mastered interviewing strategies, but I still attested to the well-known saying: "it is not what you know, it's who you know."

In 2014, after working for two months in my new part-time position, I experienced sexual assault in the work field from a physician colleague, and I ended up quitting the job after a year. In 2015, I volunteered in a medical setting and ran into another sexual harassment situation. In this case, I was stalked by a supervisor in the operations department who inappropriately monitored me. I reported the situation to my direct supervisor at that time but did not receive further support. Out of fear of retaliation and prior negative experience with the director of Human Resources, I simply quit the job as a means of speaking up for myself. I did not know that the law protects part-time workers, volunteers, and unpaid interns from sexual harassment, regardless of immigration status. In my mind, being employed to continue my professional journey was worth it, even when they paid me ten dollars an hour. I was even willing to work unpaid. As long as I was able to work in a recreational therapist position, I thought I could tolerate those disturbances at work. My mind was occupied with studying for the ATCB board exam, and I needed to complete my hours within a year because the Optional Practical Training F-1 visa only allowed me to stay for one year after graduation. At the time, I failed to sense that all of this stress was setting me up for emotional turmoil.

I Am One of Them

My practicum and internship were all completed in medical settings. The work fields were challenging yet rewarding in the sense that they prepared an art therapy intern with solid clinical training. One time while working in the psychiatric unit, I took off my coat with the badge on it before entering the group room. When I greeted the clients, I noticed that they did not acknowledge my presence for the first three minutes. As I was opening the group with a brief introduction, one of the clients finally turned his face to me and said, "Oh! Sorry, I thought you were one of the clients!" I immediately replied, "Not yet, but soon!" The atmosphere became less tense as the whole group laughed. After the group finished, I had to contact my supervisor to rescue me so I would not have to explain to each security guard that I was not a client because they would not let me through the locked doors. It was at that moment that I realized, without the nametag, I could be one of them, waiting behind the closed door, wishing to escape from the stigma.

Throughout my internship, only a few clients would notice my real name on the badge. Only three out of a hundred clients ever asked me how to pronounce my name. I enjoyed impressing my clients with the fact that I could remember all of their names and was even able to get their names right during the first session. New York is home to the most diverse array of personal names that one could find, so I received special mercy in my struggle to memorize all the clients' names. I made an effort to remember my Hungarian, Nigerian, and Russian clients' names, even with the increased difficulty in pronouncing them with my Asian accent. The forgiving thing about living in New York is that no one's accent is "perfect." Therapists could show that they care by asking their clients how they want to be addressed. It may seem insignificant, but there is a therapeutic connection when we remember each other by name, particularly in a psychiatric hospital where some clients tend to feel dehumanized.

When trying to determine my thesis topic, I was passionate about integrating my sociology background with art therapy. Narrative therapy is a great fit because therapists rely on certain sociological perspectives, such as exploring the social roles, languages, and identities of the storylines. As for the art therapy aspect, Riley and Malchiodi (2012) mentioned that art expression helps individuals gain a clearer insight into their stories, along with symbolic meanings that augment communication and the ability to problem-solve. To me, narrative therapy creates meaning using metaphors to enrich clients' stories, which can be seamless wove in the texture of expressive arts. Working with multicultural populations in medical settings and shelters for years made me conclude. In essence, a therapist's willingness to be receptive and honoring clients' extraordinary stories can generate a significant difference in their lives.

According to Michael White and David Epston (1990), people are not problems—people have problems; it was an enlightening discovery. Detaching the problem from a person thus empowers the individual to deal with the situation. The approach leads people to explore history with fresh eyes and enables them to shift the existing problems to their stories (Cobb & Negash, 2010). The belief behind this postmodern psychotherapy is that individuals are influenced, not only by their childhood experiences, but also by the broader social, cultural, political, and ethical contexts in which they live. Narrative therapy facilitates individuals to review the problems that have a profound impact on their lives from a broader point of view (Payne, 2006). I chose to believe in shapes of who I was: an international student, immigrant, foreign worker, and expatriate laborer. Yet, narrative art therapy redefined me as an individual with contributions, instead of a foreigner who does not deserve rights or benefits. As McAdams (1993) puts it, telling stories can help one attain self-realization and move toward psychological maturity. The stories I tell myself to make a difference because of the faith I hold and walk-in, leading me toward a hopeful future.

I battled several symptoms of major depression in 2013, 2015, and 2017. During my graduate studies and again while I was in my postgraduate years in the workforce, I met counselors regularly in the counseling center. It was painful to do my internship in the psychiatric unit working under pressure with limited time, handling sexual harassment, compromising my quality of life, and turning off my emotions all while undergoing my mental health crisis. I disclosed to my counselor that I severely suffered from depression, but even in that very vulnerable moment, I made jokes to conceal my anguish. It was not unusual living with depression but still managing to maintain a high daily functioning ability, to complete my duties and tasks. Internally, I was experiencing profound loss, rage, and distorted images about myself. Or I lived in the world with my "problem-saturated perspective" (White & Epston, 1990, p. 39). Upholding a daily working routine forced me to be achievement-driven. My line of work created plenty of distractions from my problems and forced me to focus on someone else's, but the depth of darkness could devour me at any time. Mentally, I was operating like a high-speed train, but once I slowed down, the train would collapse. It was unwise to chase outward success at the cost of my mental health. As a professional working in the mental health field, I confess that it was not ethical to provide services while living with mental illness, as I should have prioritized my healing first.

In My Narratives

Being an international student was a great way for me to leave my comfort zone, force me to dive into foreign territory, absorb new knowledge, and reflect on my own culture. I relocated from Long Island to several boroughs of New York to finish my studies and hunt for jobs. Every time I rush into the train stations, looking in awe at the platform overcrowded by different walks of life, I wonder what attracts other immigrants to this city. I suppose people move here to strive for all types of American dreams while I had a broken one. New Yorkers can testify how we unwittingly become aggressive, antsy, abrupt creatures; life becomes so disappointing and dissatisfying as a result of a feeling of emptiness and a fear of being uncompetitive. Nevertheless, during the toughest time in my New York life, my dedication to art therapy sustained me to trust that what I do for people, especially for the disadvantaged populations, is meaningful and essential.

Redefining my identity and rediscovering my real name has been a transformative journey. The theory of narrative therapy assisted me in examining my internalized thoughts and exploring my life experience that has been shaped by my Asian culture. In my past, when I blamed myself for not being able to obtain a full-time job, I failed to appreciate the truth: that despite many struggles, I am still a person with ethical integrity, and I have what it takes to overcome, survive, and conquer. In the fight against the stigma of mental health, I believe that we need community support and more mental health professionals with cultural competence. The Asian American population has the lowest rates in terms of medication compliance and the use of counseling resources compared to the general population nationwide (Spencer et al., 2010). My thesis research subjects were Asian Americans. The process of gathering data and interviewing different generations of Asian American immigrants helped me better comprehend how their cultural viewpoints may affect the community regarding mental health resources and its accessibility. For example, being underinsured often makes it impossible to cover the expense of mental health services, which may also correlate to a general preference in talking to family members or religious groups instead of professionals. Additionally, I found that many Asian Americans have concerns about being discriminated against for having mental health conditions, and they prefer doing physical exercises or spiritual practices to avoid medications. They also expressed experiencing adverse side effects of medicine or treatment from the clinics, which prevented them from wanting to access mental health treatment.

When I first started experiencing symptoms of severe depression, I was resistant to seeking verbal counseling services because of language barriers, also because I needed to mobilize more of my inner strength to explain what happened inside of me to the counselors. No one wants to be labeled "weak," "mentally sick," "psychotic," or "crazy." However, when my situation hit rock bottom, my extensive knowledge and experience in the mental health field provided a solid understanding to find the right support for myself. Although I felt deep shame telling my counselor that I was interning in the psychiatric unit, the first step of transformation is acceptance. I had to be honest with myself and be willing to recognize my problems. I would bring my artworks to the sessions and share them with my counselor, who focused on Cognitive Behavioral Therapy approaches. Through the counseling sessions, I gained knowledge on how to identify my triggers better, mainly that my depression was strongly associated with anger, feelings of inadequacy, a lack of confidence, and fear. My counselor did a great job of digging out my thoughts about the future, interpretations of being an international student, and all my assumptions regarding how people perceived me. On the other hand, I needed an outlet for my anger. I described myself as an anger volcano: all of the emotions hidden underneath the hurt, disappointment, and bitterness fueled the lava that could potentially initiate an explosion.

A typical workday may trigger my anger like a volcano, only because of the incident connects my deep wound of rejection. My clear memory was the time volunteering in a medical nursing home where I worked with people with dementia, developmental delays, and hearing or visually challenged. I made a cart filled with art supplies, which allowed me to go floor to floor, unit to unit to provide art sessions to the tenants. Simple Origami projects, tape art, or artwork using thick cotton yarn were my secret weapons to approaching clients. At some point, I started setting the table beside them to create a mini mobile art therapy station. My flexibility and creativity allowed me to work with a variety of clients. After volunteering for about three months, I had already received a great deal of positive feedback from clients and their families. One day, a recreation therapist in the unit, who seldom talked to me, commented, "I know why you can work with "L" (client with cerebral palsy) so well—"because she speaks so slowly, and you can learn English!" I was not quite sure what she meant, but she smiled at me, tapped me on my shoulder, and said further, "Your English is getting better!" The most frustrating part of being an immigrant worker is that my contribution to the team is often devalued as a result of my English abilities. Even the success of my therapy sessions could be viewed as a means to improve my English.

Sometimes I wonder about the future of creative arts therapy. When students start to apprehend that it is next to impossible to land a decent job that can pay the bills, even with a Master's Degree, why would they continue to pursue this type of work? Without licensure, I needed to work several jobs to sustain myself. Meanwhile, I started to develop my professional networks through various kinds of social media. One of the most productive aspects of my networking process was connecting with other volunteers. In 2015, a lawyer who volunteered in my art groups taught my colleague and me how to write a petition, which requested support for the recreation department in fighting for higher pay, raising the rate from 15 dollars per hour to 20 dollars. Eventually, we won the battle to boost the city job wages, yet I still lived hand to mouth for years.

Every day, I made art while living with depression. My art gave me the voice to express deeper layers of emotions and visualize my problems of how I perceived myself. While depression consumed me, I found myself no longer taking pleasure in making art. I used to keep art journals to manage my anxiety. In the past, I would draw an image and cut it into a circle to generate the notion that I had wrapped up my day, and I would do it daily since 2010. However, I was unable to keep up that emotional energy when I was swallowed up by my depressive pit. To me, the circle represented a sense of control. The inside of the circle signified my inner healing, which was what protected me from being affected by the world.

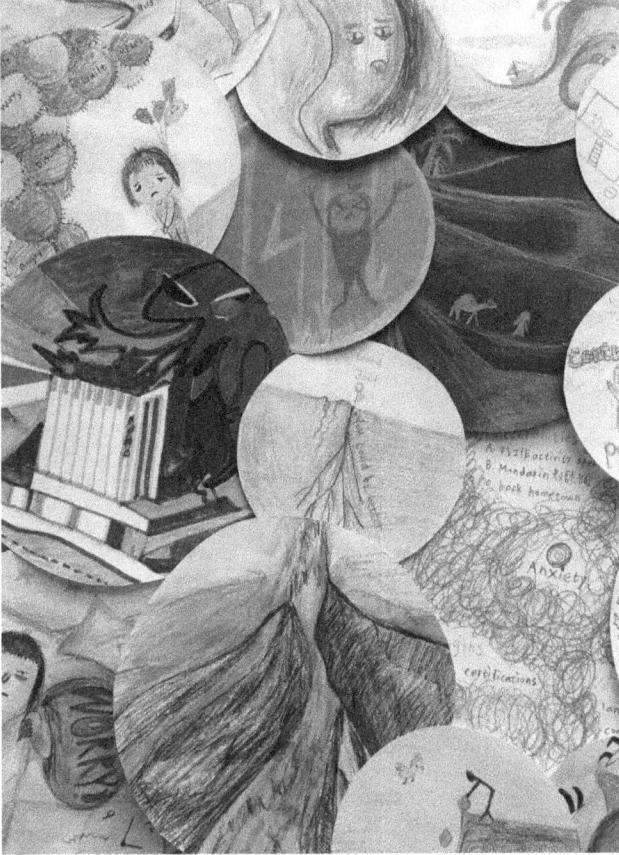

Figure 8.1 Beneath The Anger by Chia-Ling Kao.

When I started my counseling, my therapist encouraged me to revive this art routine to stimulate a feeling of aliveness again (Figure 8.1). Having a full-time job also helped me to put myself back together, as it forced myself to be productive and follow an active 9 am to 5 pm schedule every day. However, when I clocked out at the end of the day, the depression could devour me again at any time, which is why my art became the most therapeutic and valuable part of my treatment. Drawing became my language to converse with depression and anxiety. Through my art, I rediscovered that I am full of passion, knowledge, and integrity, rather than just a depressed person. To use the concept of narrative therapy, when an individual defines oneself as a whole person who has the power to manage the illness and disability, they can truly see themselves. Instead of describing the person as "psychotic" or "mentally ill," we describe the person as "living with mental illness." Rather than saying an "autistic child," we describe the child who is "living with autism." As I advocate for reducing

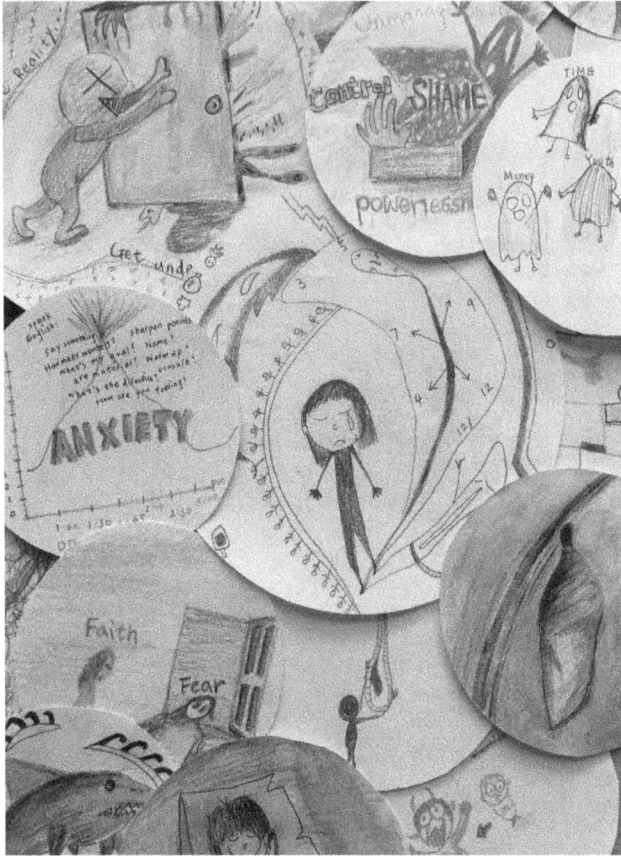

Figure 8.2 My Daily Art Journals: Drawing Emotions by Chia-Ling Kao.

the stigma of mental illness, I expect myself to be open to talking about my mental illness and maintain hope that our community will become better educated to grasp the importance of mental health support nets.

It took me years to empower myself through working with my counselors and engaging in art. During my counseling sessions, I shared narrative art therapy principles with my counselor, so we were able to use my art to discuss my core issues. In my view, narrative art therapy conceptualizes an individual's life as a story that can be presented through artistic or alternative ways. It is to examine one's difficulties with others around the person, the environment, and social systems that may dominate a person's life. Carlson (1997) integrates art materials with narrative therapy through a case study; he points out that art plays a significant role in facilitating the process of discerning the clients' problem-saturated description and visualizing their problems. Art therapy techniques clarify the notion of deconstruction in narrative therapy and enable the clients to create a new dialogue based on their internalized language (Carlson, 1997). Figure 8.3 presents the hopelessness of staying in a dark pit, facing my depression with silence. After the counseling sessions and several self-conversations, I continued to reflect on my feelings through art. Figure 8.4 refers to a process of wrestling with my depression, but knowing it was also a transformative stage of bearing a pearl.

My daily check-in drawing reflects my thoughts about self-blaming. At times, the more I drew, the more resentment I felt because I dug into my false self that tried to hide and deny the wounds I had received from others. I was not always able to sit quietly and draw something. When dealing with all sorts of emotions beneath my anger, I often had to rip off the paper several times just to calm down. Afterward, I would use the pieces of paper to

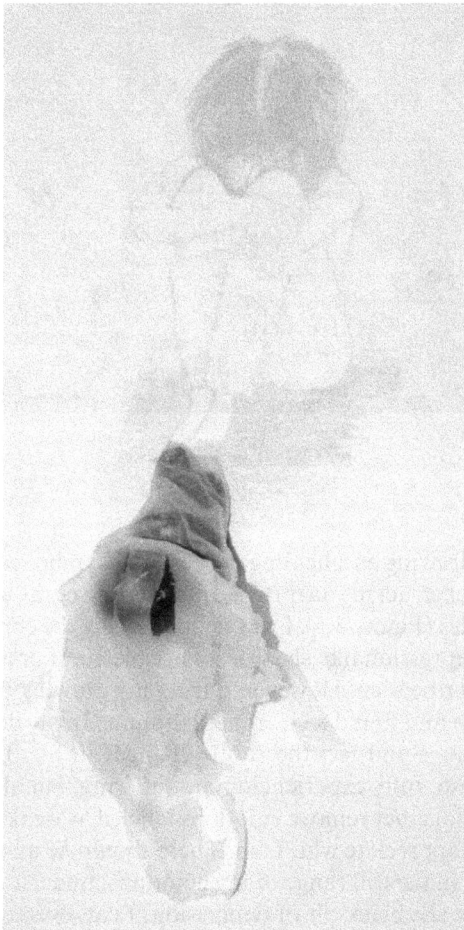

Figure 8.3 Depression and I by Chia-Ling Kao.

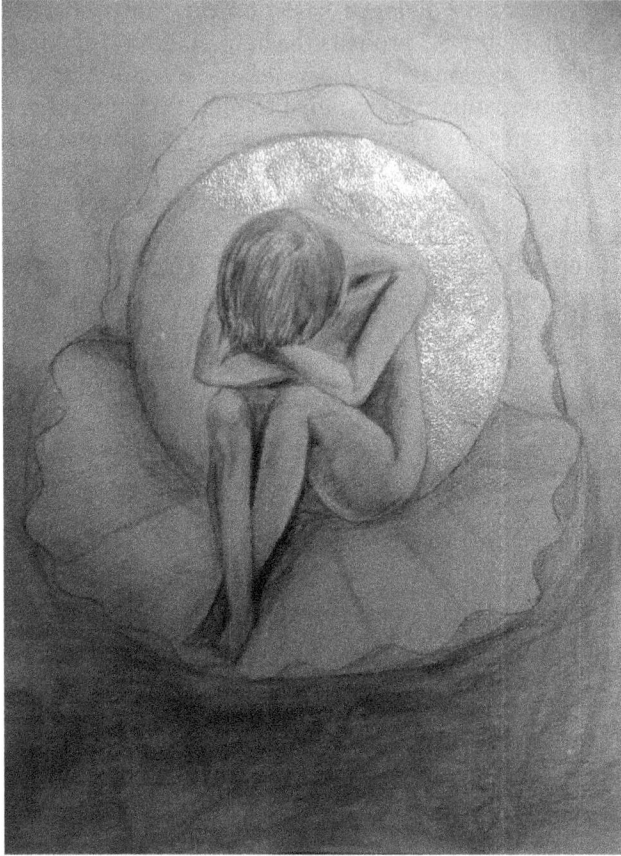

Figure 8.4 Depression and I by Chia-Ling Kao.

create another drawing as a healing process and symbolically piece myself together. To reconstruct my narratives, I started to see my weaknesses from contrasting angles (Figure 8.5). I was debilitated by the concept of wanting to destroy my depression like she was a horrible guest or a lingering ghost who should never be seen. However, during my drawing process, I talked to my depression and found a clear picture of me. In my depressive stages, I am hypersensitive and feel the subtle changes in life. I am empathetic with people's pain, fully experiencing my suffering, but also able to listen to others'. If I altogether remove emotions labeled as weak and vulnerable, I may no longer appreciate who I am. There should be an appropriate and healthy balance in the full range of my emotions, understanding that even when I return to the black pit of depression, I can overcome it. I am free when I embrace my struggles and weaknesses by realizing that they are all part of what makes me human (Figure 8.6 and 8.7).

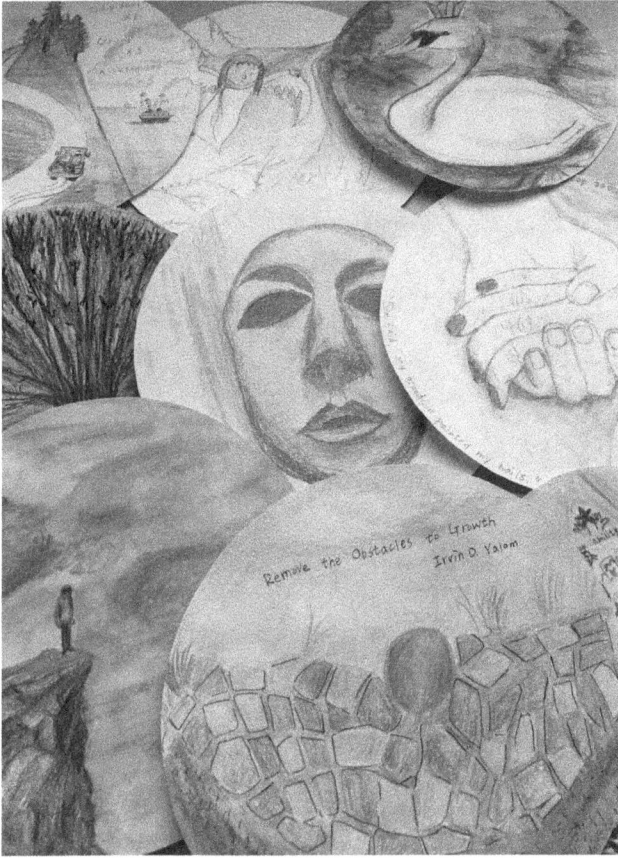

Figure 8.5 The Breakthrough Moments by Chia-Ling Kao.

The other principle of narrative therapy is to probe "the unique outcome" (White & Epston, 1990, p. 55). When it comes to combining narrative therapy with creative arts therapy, Van Der Velden and Koops (2005), who worked with survivors of war, articulated the best. They point out that narrative therapy and art therapy complement each other in helping the clients integrate their traumatic experience verbally and non-verbally. By combining story groups and art therapy, the therapeutic process frees the clients from the stereotypical framework that usually generalizes their wartime trauma. Whereas story groups provide the clients with a way to briefly review their personal history, art therapy allows clients the opportunity to extend their themes and explore details of their stories (Van Der Velden & Koops, 2005). Both narrative therapy and art therapy promote the expression of the clients' complicated feelings; these two methods work together mutually to deepen the healing effects.

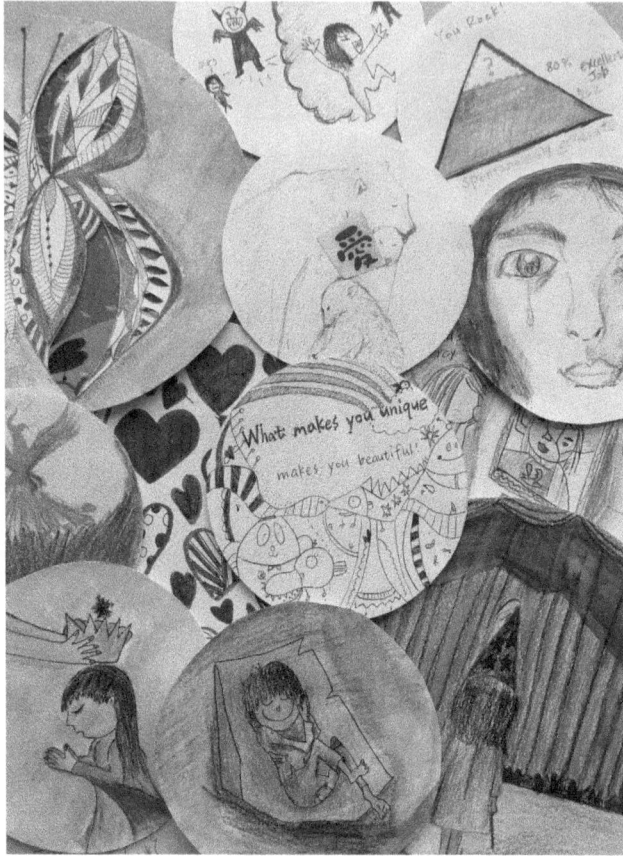

Figure 8.6 Those Little Joys And Tears by Chia-Ling Kao.

My anger and hopelessness were the underlying soil of my depression, through which I could only bear the fruit of rejection, belittlement, and oppression, especially when using "Only/Never/Always" phrases to dismiss the potential possibilities. A few of such phrases were:

> I only see White people getting favors and thriving in the art therapy field.
> No matter how hard I try, I never get management-level jobs even though I have two Master's degrees.
> I am always being picked on for my English at work.

The unique outcome of my narrative is to explore exceptions without assumptions and to develop alternative storylines that blend with past

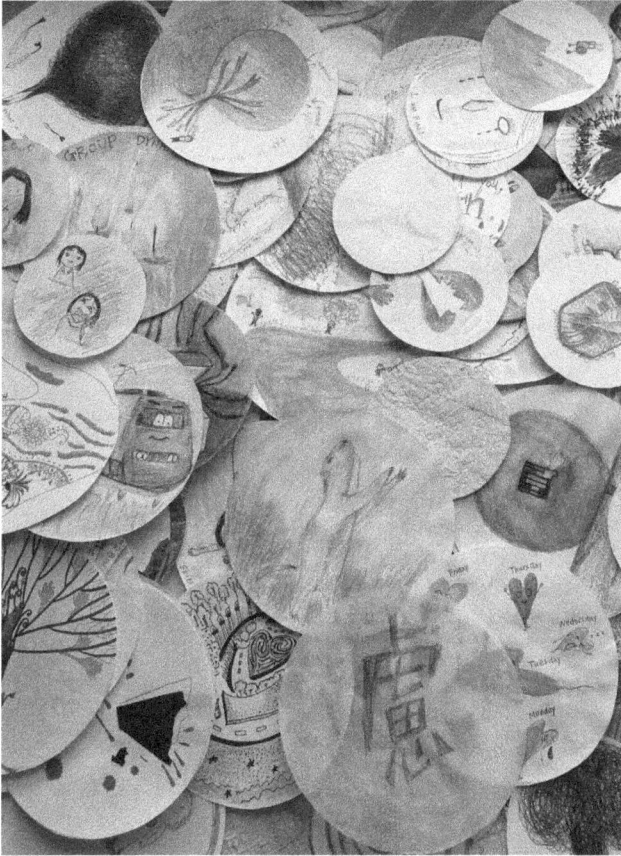

Figure 8.7 The Journey, To Be Continued by Chia-Ling Kao.

experiences for a new outcome. Therefore, my new storyline starts with: despite art therapy being a White-dominated profession at this point, I can be the one to bring the awareness and demonstrate the power of art therapy by embracing my remarkable Asian culture. Recognizing my uniqueness empowers me to reclaim my name. It is a privilege to be an art therapist working through my brokenness while experiencing the healing from art. The process has become my strength and is my passion for remaining in this field. As I gain richer experience, my ongoing delight still stems from working with varied races of clients, seeing that each minority has a voice in art, and learning how a therapist can provide a lens with multicultural sensitivity to hear. Art therapy is to honor the beauty of one's culture, the human resilience, and the uniqueness that each human can present.

References

Carlson, T. D. (1997). Using art in narrative therapy: Enhancing therapeutic possibilities. *American Journal of Family Therapy, 25*(3), 271–283.

Cobb, R. A., & Negash, S. (2010). Altered book making as a form of art therapy: A narrative approach. *Journal of Family Psychotherapy, 21,* 54–69. doi: 10.1080/08975351003618601.

McAdams, D. P. (1993). *The stories we live by: Personal myths and the making of the self.* W. Morrow.

Payne, M. (2006). *Narrative therapy: An introduction for counselors* (2nd ed.). Sage Publications.

Riley, S., & Malchiodi, C. A. (2012). Solution-focused and narrative approaches. In Malchiodi, C. (Ed.), *Handbook of art therapy* (2nd ed., pp. 103–113). Guilford Press.

Spencer, M., Chen, J., Gee, G., Fabian, C., & Takeuchi, D. (2010). Discrimination and mental health-related service use in a national study of Asian Americans. *American Journal of Public Health, 100*(12), 2410–2417. doi: 10.2105/ AJPH.2009.176321.

Van Der Velden, I., & Koops, M. (2005). Structure in word and image: Combing narrative therapy and art therapy in groups of survivors of war. *International Journal of Mental Health, 3*(1), 57–64.

White, M., & Epston, D. (1990). *Narrative means to therapeutic ends.* Norton.

9 Interweaving Art, Therapy, and Cultural Diversity

Sunhee K. Kim

Introduction

"Living in a society made up of different ethnic groups offers a paradigm for learning to participate without knowing all the rules and learning from that process without allowing the rough edges to create unbridgeable conflict" (Bateson, 1994, p. 153). According to Bateson (1994), we, as human beings, learn from our life experiences. Also, Bateson presented the idea of "peripheral vision" (p. 5), which makes it possible for us to differentiate the object from the foreground, as a way of learning different cultural points of view. For example, my experience of being placed within an American cultural context gave me several opportunities to rediscover myself and my culture. On the one hand, I was familiar with my Korean culture and customs without being conscious of it. But on the other hand, experiencing life in America made me aware of different ways of living, thinking, and interacting with others. Experiencing these discrepancies between familiar and unfamiliar helped me broaden an understanding of myself and others. I gained the peripheral vision to interweave different areas of study and cultural contexts. The concept also gave me opportunities to reflect on my personal and professional experiences.

After completing a BA degree in Education and Psychology in South Korea, I moved to the United States in 1994 to study art therapy. I was thrilled to investigate the relationship between art and psychology and how these disciplines together contribute to improving people's lives, as well as mine. The field of art therapy had not been explored in South Korea back then, and studying abroad was the only choice. Eventually, these areas—art, art therapy, education, and cultural diversity—circumscribed the fields most pertinent to my life. Their intersecting points always provide something new to challenge, explore, and express. I find it fortunate and advantageous that I was trained as a culturally sensitive and competent art therapist in multicultural communities in NYC.

Studying art therapy at New York University allowed me to learn a multicultural point of view in life. It has been a somewhat puzzling and complicated journey. For example, it was natural for me to put others' needs before my own. From collectivistic Korean culture, my conformed sense of self was weighed more in relations to others in a group. From the American context, being unique and having an individualized sense of self are highly respected. My time in the United States helped me better understand who I am as a person, re-evaluating my cultural values and assumptions. This experience has embraced me to better interact with my clients struggling with their cultural and personal conflicts. The rewarding part of this journey was finding out the self-capacity that I had not known before.

Upon completing my master's degree, I worked with various clinical settings in NYC, such as with a psychiatric creative arts therapy team, hospice care, and Alzheimer's group, a child life care team, and an immigrant social service team. With vigorous supervision along the way, my supervisors were White American, Jewish, and Asian American. I grew to be more mature and responsible—personally and professionally. My interactions with culturally diverse groups of clients, patients, families, and clinicians not only shaped and transformed my professional identity as an art therapist but also profoundly affected me as a person.

I like the word "beyond"—as art is beyond words. Art therapy is beyond the combination of art and therapy, and art therapy education goes beyond merely providing instruction and supervision for future art therapists. This chapter is about my stories as an Asian art therapist to open up further possibilities for readers to explore and expand with creative courage.

Story One: The case of Mrs. H. *(Part of this case has been published in the *Journal of Mental Health* in 2010.)

Mrs. H. was a Korean-American client in her 70s in one of the adult day health care programs in NYC. She immigrated to America in her 30s, and was widowed when I met her. Mrs. H. was diagnosed with severe depression, and had a fear of being in "therapy" and of expressing her emotions verbally (Kim, 2010). Her psychiatrist referred her to a day health care treatment center to enrich her daily life with various activities to help with her depression. Although she had good English-speaking skills, she resisted receiving any form of psychological treatment other than taking prescribed medication. From a Korean cultural perspective, I could understand her struggle: mental health such as depression is stigmatized, especially in her generation, as something that should not be discussed or something to feel ashamed to be diagnosed with. Mrs. H.'s rigid attitude towards an art "therapist" and the art "therapy" sessions at the beginning made it difficult for me to get in touch with her true self. Carl Rogers once said, "It involves the therapist's willingness for the client to be whatever immediate feeling is going on—confusion, resentment, rear, anger, courage, love, or pride. It is non-possessive caring. When the therapist prizes the client in a total rather than a conditional way, forward movement is likely" (1995, p. 116). I was able to calmly stay in contact with her even at the stage of her resistance without either pulling her or pushing her into the therapeutic alliance. I welcomed her to art "therapy" by speaking in both Korean and English. I deemed the best method of treating her would be to express empathy, supporting her inner strength, by communicating through both our mother tongue, Korean, and our second language, English. Natalie Rogers emphasized, "As companions helping to light the way, we may suggest dancing down the path, we may use guided imagery to move us along, or use visual art or sound. Whatever the method, we are on her path and she can use or refuse any of the modes we offer" (1993, p. 43). Mrs. H. was blooming with ways of expressing herself with acrylic paintings in art therapy over the time. One of special communication between us was not only the art images that she created, but her expressive writings on the back (Kim, 2010). Mostly, it was like her diary in Korean. Part of Mrs. H's writings shown on the back of her drawings translates to "Thinking of coming home from school in my childhood hometown." (Figure 9.1)

Mrs. H. had practiced and created many acrylic paintings on different sized drawing pads, sketchbooks, and canvas panels. Her favorite subjects to draw were various, such as still life, landscape, and Korean folk style painting. She preferred traditional Korean style drawing, which often contains a simple object, focalized by a large empty space left in the background. Her longing for acceptance and validation as a Korean was expressed throughout her initiation for Korean traditional style paintings

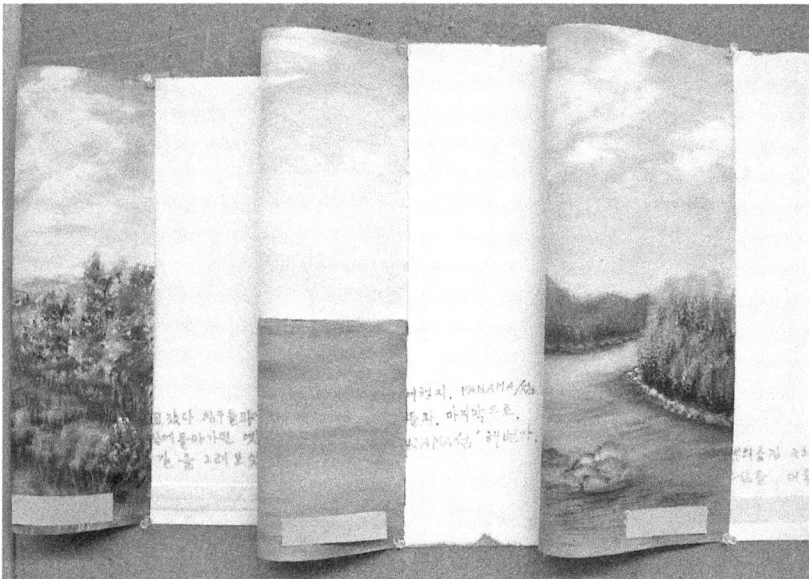

Figure 9.1 Mrs. H.'s expressive writings on the back of her paintings.

without verbal explanation. Her cultural loneliness living in a different culture, in spite of four decades of living and adjusting to fit in it, was expressed in many of her paintings. Especially in her painting, *Longing for my homeland* (Figure 9.2), she emphasized that there should be two birds on a tree, so "they are not lonely together." She said it in her fluent Korean. She did not have to explain to anyone; she connected her cultural origin through her painting, and I empathetically recognized and validated her art-making process and product, sharing cultural values.

It was interesting that she did not like abstract expressions. She seemed to prefer clear, appreciable, and unconcealed subjects over ambiguous and confusing lines, shapes, or themes for her artwork. It seemed like Mrs. H. was clearing out her depressed and anxious inner world while painting her favorite subjects. I believe that it was symbolically significant for her to express and explore her feelings and interests with such obvious subjects. Farber (1996) asserted, "Individuals are basically rational, responsible, realistic and inclined to grow" (p. 6). Throughout the art-making process and the created art products, she seemed to re-arrange and re-organize her inner world, which had not been possible with verbal expression. It was beyond her linguistic commandability, whether Korean or English, and her conscious intention to express. The relationship between Mrs. H., my Korean-American client, and myself,

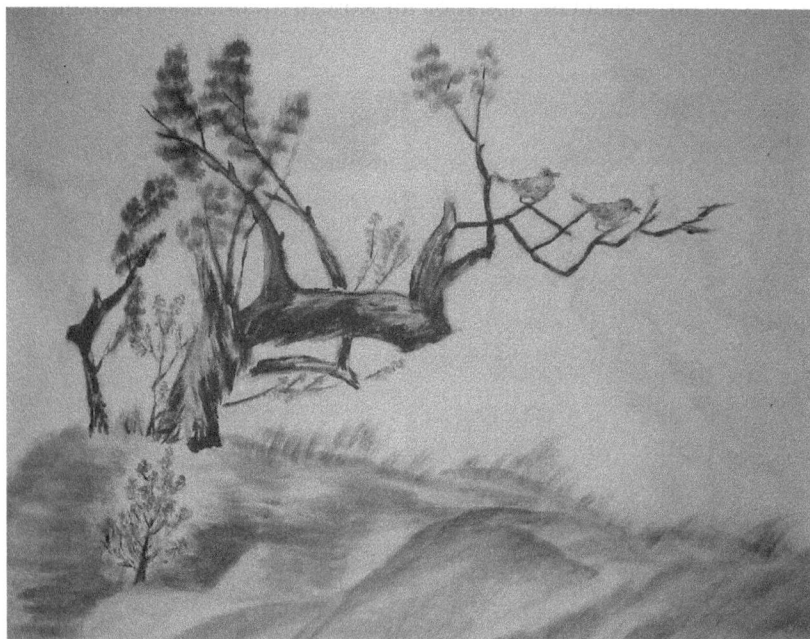

Figure 9.2 Longing for My Homeland. Acrylic painting in oriental style by a patient.

as a South Korean art therapist, went from being that of a client and therapist exchanging art images, emotions, language, and support, to one beyond the sum of art expressions, positive and negative emotions, trust, and mutual understanding of Korean culture.

It was a meaningful practice and experience for me to review the case of Mrs. H. through the lens of Korean cultural perspectives, especially dealing with negative Korean perception on treating mental health issues like depression. Through art therapy sessions together, I was confident enough to accept her resistance to "being in therapy" by knowing what it means to her as Korean, and rather support her to explore and express her inner feelings in various forms of images in her paintings without feeling shame or guilt by "staying with art" of art therapy. She has enjoyed the healing process of understanding her inner world, repressed and uncared, with the art therapist who safely participated in her journey with the shared cultural background, but without judgment.

Story Two: The Case of Mr. C. There is another case example that I would like to share here. Mr. C. was one of the art therapy group members in one of the outpatient day treatment centers in NYC. He was a White male in his early 60s, separated from his family over ten years. He came to the United States from Costa Rica to start a business and make a living by printing T-shirts, mugs, bags, etc. He was bilingual in Spanish and English, but much more fluent in Spanish than English. He was alcoholic and referred to the group art therapy to maintain and improve his well-being by participating in group activities with peers. He was losing business and he could barely manage his daily life. Fortunately, he expressed his interest in "art-making" in art therapy groups. He said, "I am an artist and designer, and that's all I am good at. Everything else is a mess!" I was running two art therapy groups on a regular basis; a Korean-American group and an English-speaking group. I offered him to experience both groups before placing him in one of the art therapy groups. Interestingly, he chose the Korean art therapy group after visiting the two groups on different days. I accepted his decision and placed him in my Korean-American group. I learned later that he felt comfortable sitting with Korean people because their mother tongue was not English just like him. We, all Korean group members and I, spoke English as a second language in the group. I wanted to unconditionally provide a supportive environment for him via active and empathetic listening (Rogers, 1995) as I did for Mrs. H. Regardless of his choice of art therapy group, I had to consider the safety of the whole group—he was poor in hygiene and there was a strong smell of alcohol with his presence. No one would sit next to him in the art room. I offered him a guideline to be in the art therapy group. "You will be welcomed and seated when you come to group sessions sober and with good hygiene. Perhaps you should consider taking a shower, changing clothes, brushing your teeth and combing your hair before coming to the program."

He was sent home the first day by the program director and warned to return the following day properly maintained to attend the program. Surprisingly enough, he showed up prim and proper and even sporting a new pair of eyeglasses. Mr. C. declared with confidence, "I need them when I draw fine lines in art class!" Since then he became an enthusiastic participant of those twice-weekly group art therapy sessions for over two years, until I had to refer him to another program due to my relocation to Korea.

It is common in NYC to encounter many groups of people from different ethnic backgrounds since NYC itself is culturally diverse. The relationship between Mr. C. and myself as a therapist had developed with more complicated cultural and symbolic exchanges through art images and creating stories on it. It was his first art image, *A Woman Enjoying Spring Breeze* (Figure 9.3) that he presented his artistic ability

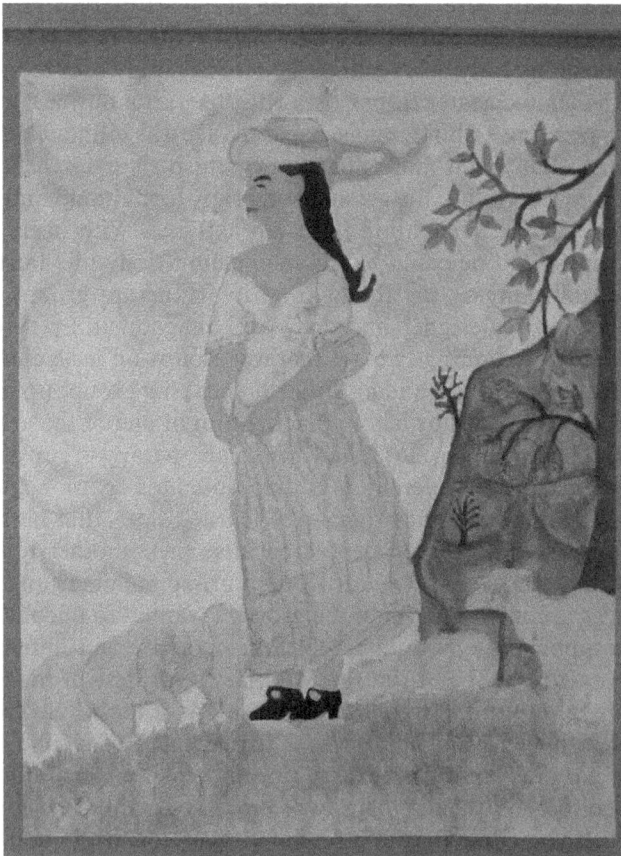

Figure 9.3 A Woman Enjoying Spring Breeze. Acrylic painting by a patient.

and willingness to become part of the art therapy group by working on one painting over several sessions working beside other members. He expressed his commitment to regaining his artistic dexterity and honing the techniques needed for his new business by both reducing his excessive alcohol consumption and by attending the art therapy program on a regular basis.

A little over three months later, a symbolically significant painting, *He Needs Help* (Figure 9.4), was completed. It depicted the relationship between a man drowning in the water, waving his two hands, and a woman in a boat named "Maria," throwing a life-saving tube close to the man in the water, where a couple of sharks are around. Mr. C. paid a lot of energy and effort on drawing the tube as visible as possible with black and white. Also, he carefully chose and controlled the black inked pen to draw the fine line connected between the hands of the woman on the boat and the tube. In the painting, the life-saving tube seemed close enough for him to grab. He made sure that everything else seemed perfect; the composition, the balance, and the story of rescue. Mr. C. proudly shared his ideas and feelings with the group art therapy participants speaking both Spanish and English, and received their attention and admiration not only for his paintings but also his positively changing attitude. To my attention, it was also an interesting representation of both the man and woman with black hair although his hair turned to grey from blond.

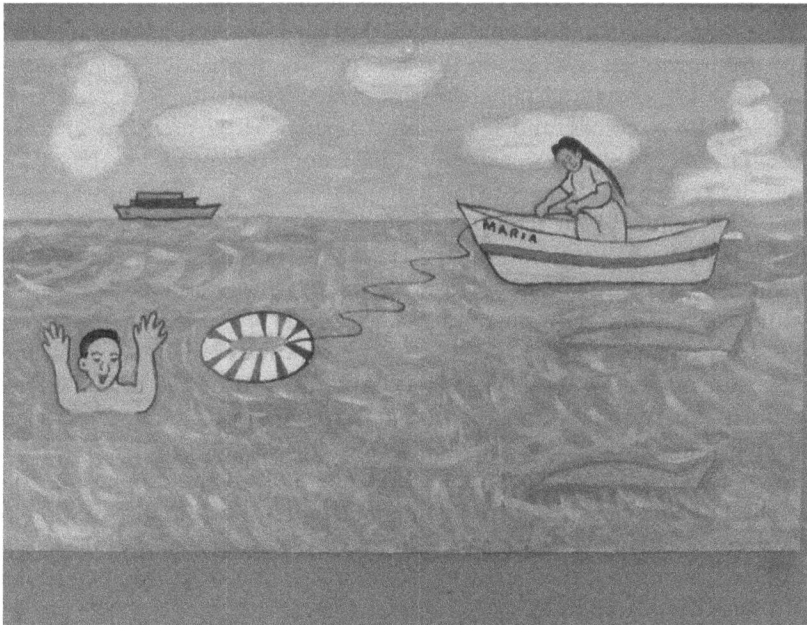

Figure 9.4 He Needs Help. Acrylic painting by a patient.

He seemed symbolically representing Asian people in his painting as a way of making a therapeutic connection to me and to the people in the group. Although the cultural backgrounds and primary languages we spoke were different, he seemed to seek and accept my help within the therapeutic alliance using art as metaphor. I was there for him not making any assumptions and judgments on him by his diagnosis, economic status, ethnicity, and verbal communication skills. However, whenever he chose his authentic themes like his hometown or his childhood memory to draw his paintings, it gave me a chance to ask questions and get to know more about him and his Costa Rican culture. Occasionally, he enjoyed teaching me some simple Spanish words and willingly learned some simple Korean from me as well.

The more Mr. C. immersed himself deeply in art making, the better his health has been improved noticeably even to all the medical staff. The recovery process was slow but for sure from heavy drinking to painting on a larger sized canvas. I would like to present two other significant paintings before coming to the conclusion on the case of Mr. C. here. Mostly, he had painted a scene where he could represent either his hometown in Costa Rica or his memory with his family, mixing colors carefully to create the similar atmosphere of his culture and the scenic view in his mind. Time to time, he asked me if I could provide him with some references such as art books, landscape calendars, postcards with famous artist paintings or photocopies of animals so he can draw and paint as real as possible. It was not my intention or instruction in art therapy to create something beautiful or realistic. Rather I have guided my art therapy group with an instruction that it is not about artistic skills or techniques. It is more about the process of creating something related to the self with lines, colors, and shapes on the paper where it can be the representation of the inner side of mind or memory. One of his acrylic paintings, however, was done copying a photograph in a calendar of Korean landscape hanging on the art room wall. Mr. C. worked very hard to build the oriental building on the right side using a ruler, a fine ballpoint pen, and a tiny brush to cover the edge. Throughout many sessions while drawing and painting on canvas, *Korea* (Figure 9.5), he had to ask me many questions about the style of the buildings in Korea, about the environment, about people and their daily life in Korea. I welcomed his curiosity about the different culture and lifestyle in Korea and returned his question to himself such as, "How was it for you to come to New York from your country, Costa Rica?", "How did you feel about planning and moving to a new environment?", and "What was it like to move alone to New York, leaving your family behind?" This was my way of interacting with my clients and their artwork no matter which language they spoke or where they came from.

My clients and I were able to connect with a shared experience that we all could relate to: leaving our home and living in a culturally different environment, where we are calling our new home. For some of the clients it was a more struggling process, and for others it was more adjusting and assimilating. Mr. C. also expressed his empathic attitude towards me working and living in the United States from Korea, speaking a different language, just like him. I acknowledged his strength expressed and explored his paintings with metaphor, representing his openness to different cultures and people. He wanted me to keep his painting, *Korea* (Figure 9.5), so whenever I feel homesick, I can imagine myself being in Korea, appreciating the Korean landscape in his artwork. I replied first with my question, "How do you deal with feelings of homesickness?", "This suggestion is based on your similar experiences?" Instead of answering, Mr. C. looked at me and nodded his head quietly. He added that he had been enjoying not only his paintings about him and his past life, but also getting ideas for making new designs for gift goods back in Costa Rica. It was not important whether or not it was realistic enough for him to plan. It was more important that he has started communicating actively with the art therapy group participants even before and after sessions, making friends with people around him beyond the language limits, and developing his identity confidently as an artist by purchasing his own art materials like high quality brushes in different sizes and shapes at Pearl Paint, a famous art store downtown in NYC, even proudly wearing beret on his head. No one had to mention his hygiene,

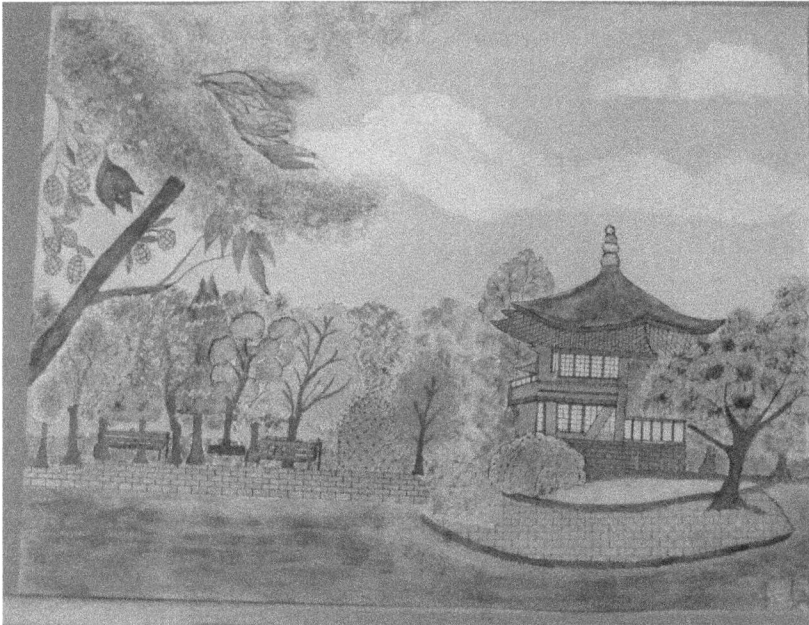

Figure 9.5 Korea, Acrylic painting by a patient.

outfit, or smells of alcohol anymore. He turned himself back as an artist that he had a dream, hope, and support to his loved ones.

It is another significant painting for Mr. C. who has suffered with alcoholism for many years. It was his idea, ironically inspired by one of photocopies of alcohol advertisements in a magazine. When preparing this painting, Mr. C. did not have any presenting alcoholic related behaviors. It did not mean that he had stopped drinking. However, he was managing his daily life, his drinking habit, and his relationship. Most of his art-making process has involved acrylic paints dealing with the adequate amount of water. He seemed to enjoy the successful moment of painting the acrylic colors on canvas without dripping by controlling the liquid. His satisfaction seemed replaced symbolically with mixing acrylic colors and water from mixing drinks. One action is healthy enough to be encouraged and acknowledged by others, and the other is negatively affected to his health and life causing many relational problems. Not like what his painting says, "NO DRINK," (Figure 9.6). Mr. C. has struggled with alcohol continuously. However, he was under control not by outside force or pressure, but by himself, gaining a sense of control, of satisfaction, and of success throughout art-making and sharing the process and the product with significant others to him. Mr. C. had reduced his expenses on drinking. I was reported by his social worker that he rather saved more money to purchase good and newest art materials than

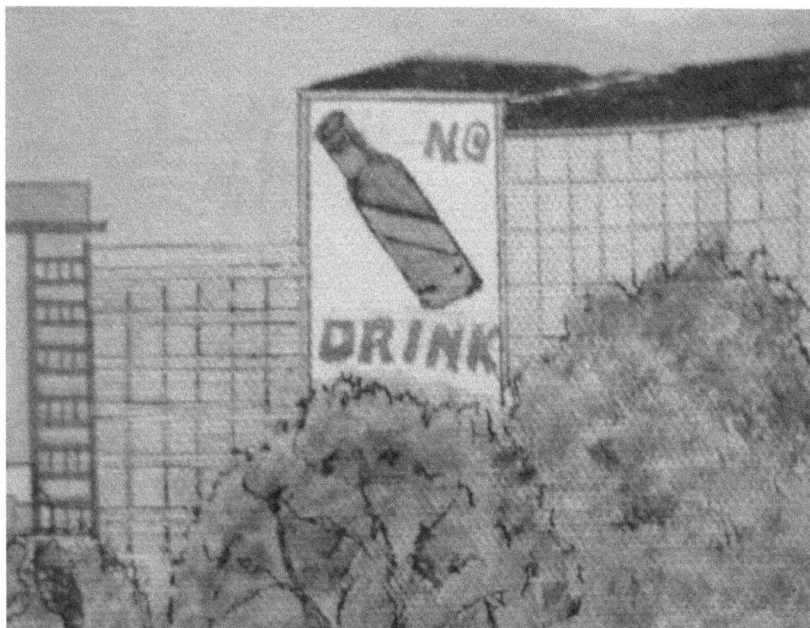

Figure 9.6 *No Drink*, Acrylic painting by a patient.

buying alcohol bottles and cans. He had spent more time either shopping at the art store, Pearl paint, by taking subways, or working at home on his own canvas stretched on a wooden frame. Almost two years of his working-in-progress was supported not only by many staff and art therapy group members including me as therapist, but most importantly, by his ability to contact and embrace his true self inside. I believe it seemed safe enough for Mr. C. to navigate his inner self with the therapeutic alliance we had built together over the time, despite many different aspects such as culture, language, age, and gender.

At last, I am very excited to present Mr. C.'s final artwork from the group art therapy. It was when we had to consider terminating the art therapy group in six month or so. Due to a financial situation, the whole program had to be transferred to other institutions in NYC, and I had to refer my art therapy group participants to the places where they have similar art therapy programs as long as possible. It has not been easy, rather difficult, for me as a therapist to go through the termination process, especially with long-term clients like Mr. C., who heavily rely on the art and its dynamic with the process and the therapeutic relationship. It has involved many sessions to consider and discuss the closure of the art therapy group together. Some were in denial that they would not think until the day actually comes. The others were a bit upset but wanted to consider some of the options that they were left with. Mr. C. seemed very disappointed at first but responded pretty calm over the course. He had accepted the reality and started talking about his plan: visiting other programs to participate and creating his last artwork as a masterpiece during the rest of the art therapy group sessions. I started exploring with Mr. C. in the group about his termination plan; what "masterpiece" meant for him, in which way he wanted to prepare and set up the art material for it, and if there were anything he would like to ask for me or for the program. It did not take long for him to ask, "Would it be possible to get a really big canvas which stands itself? It will be my last painting here and I will paint my masterpiece finally!" I knew Mr. C. did not really expect for me or the program buying such expensive art materials for him. Intuitively, I thought of my own 4' by 4' size canvas panel. It was my personal artwork originally done with acrylic paint, which I titled, *Sky Has No Borders* (Figure 9.7), about three years before I met Mr. C. in the art therapy group. It was created along with my grieving process of my loving father, who passed away suddenly. I had not shared my personal story then with Mr. C. nor the art therapy group. While considering giving my own canvas painting to him, I asked whether or not he was interested in using my artwork panel for his final artwork by showing him a photo first. I wanted to give him a choice and would like him to consider the huge size of canvas, which he had never worked on before. I thought my sky painting would be a good background for his painting so he would not be challenged with empty white space which was too big to

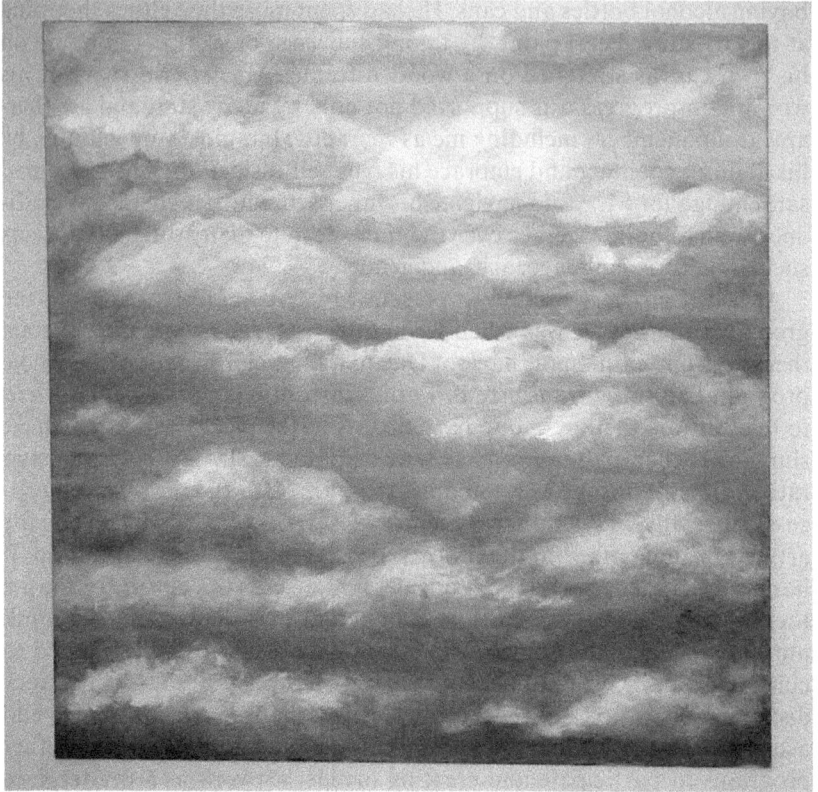

Figure 9.7 Sky Has No Borders. Acrylic painting by Sunhee K. Kim.

cover by himself within the time frame we had until termination. When he saw the photo of my canvas, he was surprised and excited, "I don't have to paint my sky here. It is the kind of sky that I like and it will create my masterpiece here! Let me see what I can do. You don't change your mind, Ok? Just bring it to me as soon as possible!"

I had to explain this special occasion to the art therapy group and received the entire members' agreement without any hesitation. I had never given my artwork to my client to work on before. I felt guilty having to leave him at the very important period of his progress when he transformed from a heavy alcoholic to an artist who could create his own paintings with various art materials. I was returning to my home country leaving him in NYC, knowing how much he missed his home himself. I wanted to leave my meaningful artwork, which was created when I was left alone. I do not know whether or not it was a cultural gesture as a Korean art therapist; I do not know whether it was a professional gesture as a therapist. However, I have absolutely no regrets that I had provided it to Mr. C. then for the following reason; it was a critical time for him to "flow" with his restored identity—a sober artist—and I wanted it to be continued without interruption despite the expected termination of the group art therapy program at the center. He was still in need of some external support and connection to rely on. His self-confidence has been built stronger but should not be shaken again. He had spent over five months to complete his "masterpiece," *My New York City,* (Figure 9.8). I could not help but compare it with his previous artwork, *He needs help* (Figure 9.4), depicting a man drowning in the water. The structure of the two images contains similar elements; the sky and the water. However, it cannot be missed on his final painting to see the transformation of his symbolic representation of himself, his environment from, and his relation to the world. It seemed to be displaced a man seeking help in the guise of the Statue of Liberty representing freedom; sharks in water as various ships; the boat "Maria" as the George Washington Bridge firmly spans across the whole canvas. Look at all the vehicles on the bridge. He worked very hard to paint them with all different designs in detail. He has developed fine motor skills over the time of painting and controlled his shaky hands due to alcoholism almost perfect for his "masterpiece."

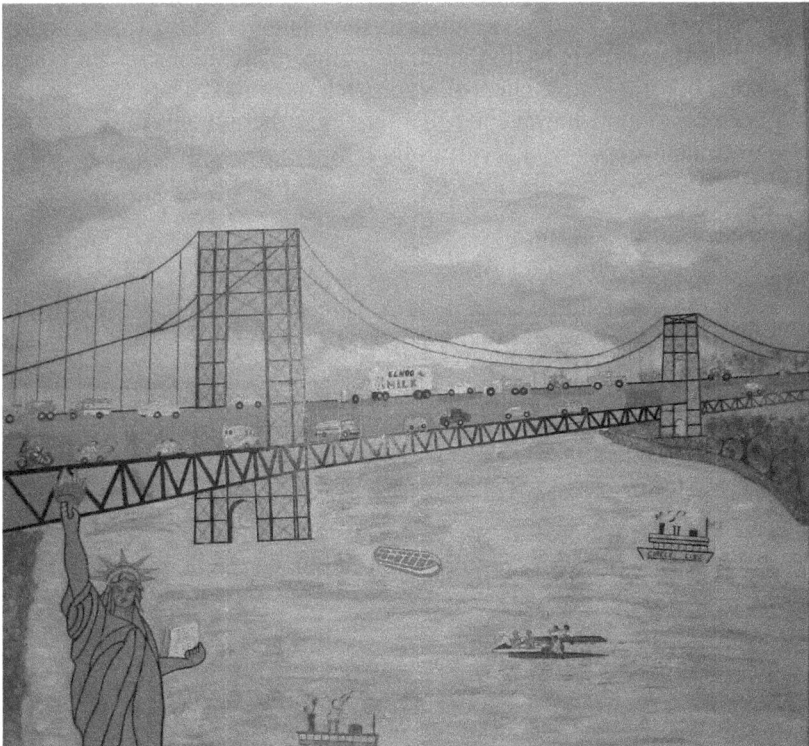

Figure 9.8 My New York City. Acrylic painting by a patient.

Most of all, I had never seen him with such excitement to explain to the group how busy and active the people were on the road and on the river in his painting. The art therapy group shared together the whole change, challenge, and growth that Mr. C. had gone through, and moreover, the last day of his completion of his "masterpiece." He seemed deeply moved and grateful by saying, "Well, I didn't know if I could really do this. It was not easy, but I enjoyed it, you know. I feel good and very sad that it is time to say goodbye." It was an unforgettable moment for all of us then and so far to me.

Art becomes a pathway to access emotions and creativity. During the art-making, it is possible to lose yourself somewhere in the imagined world, but safely, you return because you are not lost. You are in real contact with your genuine self, the process of creating your world upon the given space—the canvas or the paper—you flow through your inner self kindly and patiently. With such self-motivated, creative energy, you can immerse yourself into even difficult emotions and experiences that eventually give a sense of accomplishment and mastery. There were many moments that we as a person existed true to each other in the space beyond the words, carrying the hope beyond we can anticipate. My deepest gratitude and appreciation go to my clients, Mrs. H. and Mr. C., who eventually transformed me as much as they changed along their journey to healing through art. With their trust in me, my relationship with them has gone beyond simple client-therapist relationships. They have helped me become a more humble art therapist, art therapy educator, and an open-minded person who is culturally sensitive.

References

Bateson, M. (1994). *Peripheral visions: Learning along the way*. Harper Collins.

Farber, B. A. (1996). Introduction. In B. A. Farber, D. C. Brink, & P. M. Raskin (Eds.), *The psychotherapy of Carl Rogers: Cases and commentary* (pp. 1–14). The Guilford Press.

Kim, S. (2010). A story of a healing relationship: The person-centered approach in expressive arts therapy. *Journal of Creativity in Mental Health*, *5*(1), 93–98.

Rogers, C. (1995). *A way of being*. Houghton Mifflin.

Rogers, N. (1993). *The creative connection: Expressive arts as healing*. Science & Behavior Books.

10 Intracultural Practice for Asian Art Therapists

"Are You One of Us, or Are You One of Them?"

Miki Goerdt

Introduction

In the art therapy field, the phrase diversity and cultural competency generally refer to the intercultural practice, which is defined by working with clients whose background differs from therapists' their own. Intracultural practice, which is defined as working with clients from the same racial/ethnic group of the therapist (Shulman, 2015), is another aspect of clinical practice that requires cultural competency. Intracultural practice for minority art therapists brings different sets of challenges from Caucasian-to-Caucasian intracultural practice. However, these challenges for minority therapists are rarely discussed in professional training and research in the art therapy field. Shulman (2015) describes that intracultural practice comes with "more difficult and often painful" (p. 54) issues than intercultural practice. Some challenges mentioned in this chapter may be everyday experiences of minority individuals in their intracultural communication, not just Asians. However, this chapter is focused on encounters between Asian therapists and Asian clients. The purpose of this chapter is for art therapists to gain an understanding of the key elements to examine in intracultural practice, particularly in the interactions between Asian art therapists and Asian clients. This chapter also is intended to aid Asian art therapists' exploration of their identity as an art therapist.

Asian Clients' Preference to See An Asian Therapist

In my private practice, over half of my clients identify themselves as Asian or minority, including Japanese, Korean, Chinese, Thai, and Singaporean. In the initial session with them, I usually have asked how they selected me as their therapist. Some of them chose me because of the language I speak (Japanese) because they cannot effectively communicate in English. Many of them say they wanted a therapist who is the same race/ethnicity as them. They told me, "I thought you'd understand where I'm coming from." "You would know 'the Asian way,' and I don't have to explain to you." "I thought we'd have something in common." It's clear that my appearance meant something to them, and they came in with a set of assumptions about how I can relate to them. Studies have indicated that minority clients prefer seeing therapists of the same racial group (Cabral & Smith, 2011), and Asian-American clients tend to see Asian therapists as more credible and similar to them (Meyer et al., 2011).

The perceived similarity with therapists can create an illusion of understanding and a sense of security (Meyer et al., 2011). Empathy and a sense of security are elements that clients in psychotherapy often seek. Thus it is not surprising that clients try to find someone who is visually similar to them. In addition, the broader societal beliefs and racial assumptions influence minority individuals' decision to see minority therapists. According to Fors (2018), there is a common assumption in the mainstream culture that minority people would automatically understand each other because of the shared status of being in a subordinate group. Fors (2018) describes that this untrue assumption produces the minority individuals' hope and desperation to experience the automatic understanding between minority therapists and them. The study by Chang and Yoon (2011) also illustrated the minority clients' tendency to avoid discussing racial/cultural issues with their White therapists because they felt White therapists could not understand important aspects of their experiences. One can easily assume that this avoidance may result in the minority client's inability to fully explore the sense of self or not fully benefitting from the therapy. Another study also indicates that White therapists feel uncomfortable with discussing racial and cultural issues in sessions (Utsey et al., 2005).

The assumption that the White therapists would not understand minority individuals' experience can create pressure for minority individuals to explain themselves when they are in front of a White therapist. King (2018) points out that minority individuals in the United States feel responsible for educating White people about experiences of what it's like to be a minority. "Belonging to a subordinated group and mentalizing the perspective of majority persons who are not always returning the favor can be suffocating" (Fors, 2018, p. 129). The responsibility to facilitate understanding in White individuals/therapists is a tiring task for minority individuals, especially when they are seeking services to work on psychological distress such as depression, anxiety, and loss. For a minority individual, seeing a minority therapist means he/she is free from feeling this sense of responsibility. In addition, minority clients may also seek minority therapists to reduce the risk of experiencing negative judgment from White therapists. Vasquez (2007) describes that minority clients may be more susceptible to a sense of shame due to the history of oppression, and they may present more sensitivity toward White therapists' rejection, negative judgment.

Key Elements in Intracultural Encounters Between Asian Clients and Asian Art Therapists

Research shows that Asian Americans were more likely to stay in treatment when they worked with an Asian-American counselor (Takeuchi et al., 1995). However, having the same race/ethnicity is not a guarantee for building an effective therapeutic relationship. Studies on the effect of a racial match between clients and therapists have inconsistent results (Flaskerud & Liu, 1991; Fiorentine & Hillhouse, 1999; Gamst et al., 2004; Wu & Windle, 1980). The expectation of the Asian clients' part to have their Asian therapist's full understanding of their cultural background may result in disappointment and painful experience in some encounters for both clients and therapists.

Several factors complicate the relationship between an Asian art therapist and an Asian client:

Asian as a diverse group of individuals. The racial group called "Asian" is a diverse. U.S. Census Bureau (2000) recognized 24 ethnicities among individuals under the group name of Asian Americans. Within this group, there were multiple cultures and languages. This means the racial match of an Asian client with an Asian therapist does not expect a cultural match.

Acculturation orientation of both parties. The same race does not mean the same orientation of acculturation in both parties. Acculturation is the process of culture change and adaptation that occurs when individuals with different cultures come into contact (Gibson, 2001). Various models exist to conceptualize acculturation, as discussed in LaFrambiose et al. (1993). For this chapter, I will use the acculturation model introduced by Berry (1980) as a framework. It is a bilinear model of acculturation whereby it is possible and most desirable for an individual to adhere to both her/his culture of origin and dominant culture. In Berry's (1980) model, the acculturation of individuals is described by four orientations: integration, assimilation, separation, and marginalization. Integration happens when an individual maintains adherence and proficiency in both the indigenous and dominant cultures. Assimilation occurs when an individual feels more comfortable with the dominant culture and has little association with the indigenous culture. Separation happens when an individual maintains adherence to the indigenous culture but does not adapt to the dominant culture. Marginalization happens when an individual rejects both the indigenous and dominant cultures. In intracultural interactions with clients, the Asian therapist may be in one orientation and Asian clients in another. When two parties are not in the same orientation of acculturation, clients may feel they may not be understood (e.g., "My therapist is too Americanized."). Acculturation differences may also make the therapist feel pressured to be "Asian-enough" to be accepted by Asian clients.

In my practice, clients, especially Japanese clients with whom I share the cultural origin, are eager to find out my acculturation level. They often ask how long I lived in the United States, which city in Japan I am from, how often I go back to Japan, and if I miss Japan. It is as if they are saying, "You look like me. Do you think like me? I hope you do. You are one of us, right? Or are you more like one of them (Americans)?" Many of these Japanese clients in my practice are immigrants who have resided in the United States for a few years, and their ties to their home country remain strong. Many of them are in the separation orientation described in Berry's (1980) acculturation model. It is my experience that Asian immigrant clients with the separate orientation of acculturation are often unfamiliar with the role of a therapist. As a result, such clients may try to relate to their Asian therapists in the same manner that they relate to other Asians they encounter in the community. This may manifest as clients' actions of offering gifts, bringing food for therapists, providing advice on personal matters when the therapist is younger than them, and ask about the therapist's home country and family. Wong et al. (2007) found Asian-American clients tended to stay in treatment longer and were more satisfied when education on therapeutic processes and the purposes of interventions were provided. Providing them some explanations on how a therapeutic relationship differs from friendship gives them some structure in the relationship with the therapist.

In addition to clarifying the role of the therapist, it can be helpful to provide explanations to Asian clients on how assessments and treatment modalities such as art therapy serve the specific purpose in relation to treatment goals. Providing such structure and education may help Asian clients to distinguish their expectations on a therapist from one they would on another Asian in the same room. This can be the foundation of building a trusting relationship despite acculturation differences. The assessment of the client's acculturation orientation determines how much direct communication, such as explanations and education, should be provided to create a sense of comfort in Asian clients. Less acculturated Asians (i.e., ones who associate themselves more with the indigenous culture) tend to see therapists with direct communication style more satisfying and credible (Kim & Park, 2015). Li and Kim (2004) also found that Asians who adherer to Asian cultures prefer direct counseling style, which is characterized by the use of the therapist's skills, including choosing the goal, clarifying the problem, interpreting, conveying of information, directing clients' behaviors, and making suggestions.

Asian art therapists' sense of obligations to their communities. Lack of culturally and linguistically appropriate services for Asian Americans contributes to underutilization of mental services, along with other reasons such as stigma and shame about mental illnesses (Kim-Goh et al., 2015). My circumstance is not an exception to this nation-wide problem;

I am one of a few therapists who speak Japanese in the Northern Virginia region. Because only a limited number of therapists are proficient in the language to serve Japanese clients in my area, I feel pressured to serve when they contact me. When I tell them my schedule cannot accommodate, I know this means they most likely have no other option and may end up not receiving therapy. This sense of pressure was also reported by other Japanese therapists who attend a quarterly peer supervision group in my area.

History has plenty of examples of the unmet needs of minority groups by mainstream society. Minority individuals rely on their group identity to support and heal from the impact of racial oppression and internalized oppression (King, 2018). Studies have found that collectivism is one of the main characteristics of Asian culture (Kim et al., 1999; Kim & Omizo, 2005; Sue & Sue, 2003). Collectivism, an ideology that emphasizes the unity of the group over individuals, comes with the demand for cooperation from the group members (VandenBos, 2007). From this perspective, it is common and expected for Asian therapists to feel obliged to an Asian client's request for help. Often Asian communities function like a small village, where everyone knows everyone. It is not uncommon that Asian therapists and Asian clients may exist in the same close-knit community, sharing friends and acquaintances. Like the issue of acculturation level difference, Asian therapists' sense of obligation to their communities complicates intracultural encounters. One can speculate that some Asian clients would feel disappointed when "the obligation" of being a member of the community is not honored by an Asian therapist from their community.

The Dissonance Between Western-Centered Theories and Asian Cultures in Art Therapy Education

Western psychology theories often focus on the establishment of self and the empowerment of the individual as a treatment goal. However, much like other cultures of minority groups, Asian culture is of collective culture. According to Ford et al. (2015), individuals in collectivistic cultures pursue happiness through their relationships with others. Asians define themselves as a member of the group, and group cohesion is valued more than the establishment of self-identity. As a result, how other people see them is very important to them. In the Asian cultural perspective, the self only exists as a part of the group, and the group identity dominates more than the self identity. Many Asian clients who come into my office see their focus on other's perceptions about them as negative. They say, "Why do I worry about what other people think so much?" "Why can't I pay attention to myself and my own needs more? I must not value myself enough." They complain about their lack of assertiveness and not having opinions of their own. For Asians living in the United States, their traditional way of living looks as if they failed to form a strong sense of individuality when they compare themselves to individuals in the dominant Western culture.

Therapists can help reframe clients' negative views on this structural difference of Western and Eastern societies and help them to see that it is a result of cultural differences; the Western way is not better than the Eastern way. With this understanding, therapists and clients can explore how clients want to think of themselves. Clients can then aim at finding a way to balance what their traditional Asian value system influence compare with them and what the dominant Western culture portrays as "healthy." Without addressing their negative perception about their own culture, the therapist may end up leading Asian clients to work on acquiring what the dominant culture portrays as a "healthy sense of self." This puts clients at risk for distancing themselves from the traditional culture unintentionally.

Not only the dissonance of Western psychological theories with Asian cultures, but there is also a fundamental difference in approaches to problem-solving between East and West. De Vaus et al. (2018) describes that Easterners and Westerners process negative emotions differently because Eastern thoughts tend to be holistic and Western thought analytic. The holistic approach of the East is not addressed in formal education in the West. This may result in leaving Asian therapists with a toolbox borrowed from the Western culture to treat their people unless they work on exploring how they can weave the Western approach into the Asian cultures.

Therapists are taught in graduate programs and training to build an egalitarian relationship with a client. However, Asian clients typically see a therapist as a credible and authority figure because a hierarchical structure is emphasized in Asian cultures (Kim-Goh et al., 2015; Nipponda, 2012). The Western therapeutic approach may make Asian clients uncomfortable, especially when they are in the traditional or transitional orientation of the acculturation. At the beginning of my practice, I strongly encouraged my Asian clients to see me as a partner rather than an authority. I corrected them when they called me "Sensei (teacher/doctor/an authority figure)" and asked them to call me by my first name. Now I practice differently. I no longer correct them if they prefer to call me Sensei. I often accept them seeing me as an authority figure if this puts them more at ease to engage in therapy. Asian clients also expect that therapists take the lead in structuring sessions and make the treatment goal clear (Substance Abuse and Mental Health Services Administration, 2014). This means it is more culturally appropriate to provide specific art directives instead of a free drawing task or open studio style of art therapy. I provide a fair amount of psycho-education and then inquire about their reactions to what they hear from me.

For Asian art therapists, the dissonances between East and West in their art therapy education can impact their clinical practice significantly, creating a divide between the personal self and the professional self. Some Asian therapists/students in graduate programs may hesitate to challenge authority figures such as professors to address this dissonance. Even if they question, professors may not be equipped to answer the questions of how to integrate the two very different cultures into a culturally competent art therapy practice. When I asked for guidance on boundary issues with Asian clients in my graduate course to a White art therapy professor, she responded, "What do you think? You may be more knowledgeable on this topic. How is it handled in your culture?" This type of response comes with a possible consequence of assigning Asian art therapy students to the responsibility of exploring appropriate clinical actions on their own.

Lack of support and opportunities to question and explore the dissonance may increase the likelihood of molding Asian art therapists as "Western therapists in the Asian skin" upon graduation. When they face Asian clients in clinical work, they may feel lost as to how to integrate what Western education taught them into what they know from their Asian backgrounds. Given the fact that art therapy is a predominantly White profession (Elkins & Deaver, 2013), Asian art therapy students have few opportunities to consult and explore with other Asians in the same field regarding the dissonance mentioned above. Aside from mandala drawing and mindfulness, much of Eastern traditions would be left out of the formal art therapy education. This contributes to the creation of many unanswered questions that need exploration and clarification when an Asian art therapist enters into the workforce.

Language/Communication Barriers

Lastly, communication and language barriers can exist between Asian art therapists and Asian clients, even if they are from the same country. When Asian therapists study counseling in English speaking counties such as the United States, it is often difficult to describe psychological concepts or articulate feelings and thoughts with wording typically used in counseling in the Asian languages (Kim-Goh et al., 2015). Technical terms and phrases unique to psychology are beyond the daily conversation level of communications. This means Asian art therapists would be expected to spend time familiarizing themselves with specific counseling terms and phrases in their Asian language if they plan to use it with clients.

Self-Awareness as An Asian Art Therapist

Because there is no right or wrong answer that fits in every intracultural encounter, Asian therapists' self-awareness would be the most useful tool to determine how to proceed to build a trusting relationship with an Asian client. In speaking of cross-cultural practice in art therapy, Hocoy (2002) recommended art therapists to become aware of one's own cultural lens, aware of the assumptions and values on which theory and technique in art therapy are based, and examine our biases about other cultures. American Art Therapy Association (2011) also issued the statement to stress the importance of self-awareness and sensitivity to one's cultural heritage, if one is to be a culturally competent art therapist. Examining a view about cultures, especially their own culture in addition to other cultures such as the dominant culture, can help Asian art therapists to be able to distinguish personal reactions (which often leads to counter-transference) from clinical insights (which leads to effective treatment) during sessions with Asian clients. The following art directives are designed to explore and raise self-awareness of Asian art therapists' cultural identity as well as reactions in intracultural encounters:

Exercise #1: Use a 12 × 18 drawing paper. Fold in half. One side describes your traditional culture. The other side describes the dominant culture. Include representation of yourself (e.g., figure, symbol, an animal) somewhere on the paper.
Reflective questions:

1   What feelings arise as you look at each side?
2   Which side was easier to create? Which one was more difficult?
3   Were there elements that you were unsure of which side to place?
4   Which side was "the representation of you" placed? How do you make sense of the placement?
5   Explain how two sides relate to each other.
6   What acculturation orientation (assimilation, integration, separation, and marginalization) do you observe in your art? What do they mean to you?

Exercise #2: Create an image of how your Asian clients see you. This can be about one particular client or your clients as a group.
Reflective questions

1   What are adjectives to describe the images? Let's make a list.
2   Out of these adjectives, which ones are consistent with how you see yourself? Is there a difference in how your clients see you and how you see yourself in terms of cultural identity and acculturation orientation?
3   What created the difference seen in the question (2)?
4   How does the difference seen in the question (2) affect your relationship with the client?

A Personal Reflection

When I conducted self-reflection through the first exercise, I found myself in the middle of the paper (Figure 10.1). I am looking back toward my traditional culture (right side), but my body faces the dominant culture side (left side). I feel guilty for portraying my traditional culture the way I did in this drawing, dark and haunting. I left Japan when I was 18 years old, and I lived in the United States for over 20 years. The majority of my time in the United States was spent in predominantly White communities without much diversity or Japanese people to interact with. In this drawing, I mostly see myself as someone in the assimilation orientation of acculturation. I am more comfortable with the dominant culture. I became this way because I had to assimilate to survive in the places where my traditional culture seemed too foreign. Many lacked an understanding of what it means to accept differences, and this translated into their actions of discrimination and stereotyping. I sense kindness and warmth toward the dominant culture side despite uncomfortable experiences because "becoming more like Americans" in a predominantly White community meant more opportunities, more friends, success, and possibilities. As I look at my drawing, I recognize a part of me who wants to move to the integration orientation: the figure is placed in the middle, and her eyes are looking at the direction of traditional culture. Part of me wants to re-establish and maintain the connection to the traditional side, wanting to remember what's there. When I look at the side of the traditional culture of this drawing, sadness comes up. I feel constricted by

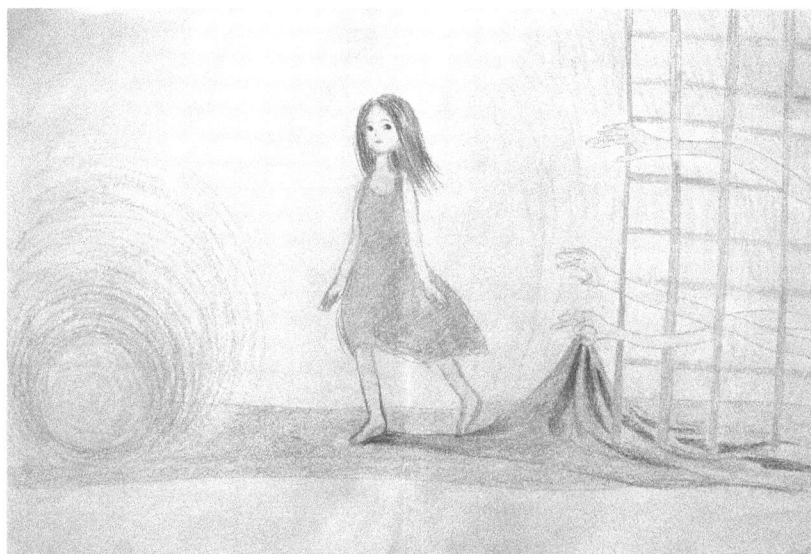

Figure 10.1 Cultural Identity. Drawing by Miki Goerdt.

rules, feel responsible for caring for others, but couldn't, and feel guilty to leave my loved ones behind. It is the guilt I felt when I left my home country, and it is the guilt I feel when I say to Japanese clients, I have no openings in my schedule. As I look at this drawing, I realize that I have some work to do. I want to be at home with two cultures that form who I am. I identify a sense of guilt and sadness that is waiting to be processed. Two sides do not interact much in this drawing. Two sides look divided by me as if I am a wall that prevents one side from contacting the other. Suddenly another realization hits me. Instead of becoming a wall that divides the two sides, I am capable of becoming the space where two sides interact harmoniously.

For the second exercise, I decided to explore how I think my Asian clients, especially Japanese clients, see me (Figure 10.2). I drew myself on a recliner in my office, sitting up straight with a pair of glasses. The words

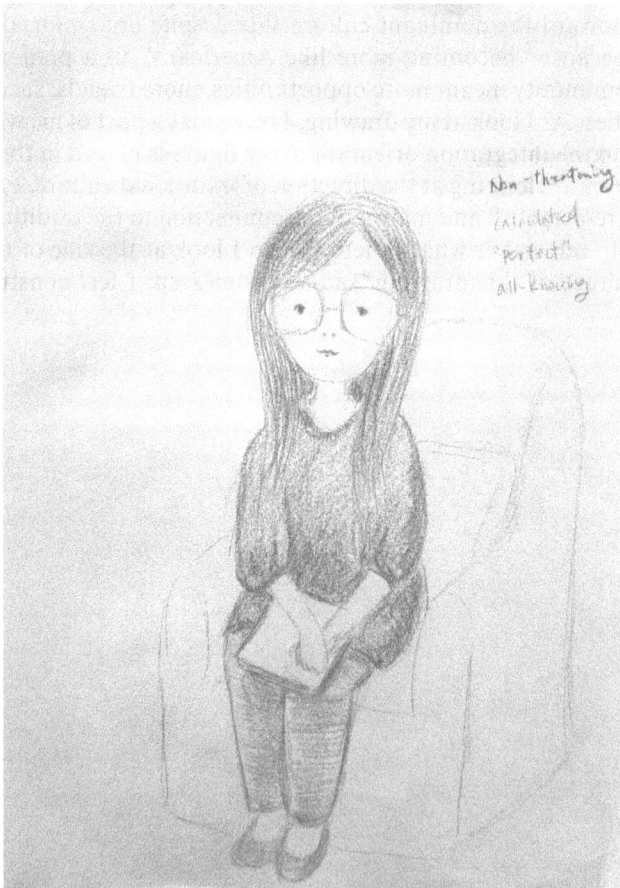

Figure 10.2 Self-portrait. Drawing by Miki Goerdt.

that come to my mind with the image are non-threatening, calculated, all-knowing, and perfect. I think to myself, "I am none of these things in real life." I think of some clients who call me "Sensei," even after I inform them they can call me by my first name. The word Sensei means a teacher, and it also means a doctor. It signals the authority. They see me as a guide with the authority to solve problems for them.

The self-awareness through this exercise helps me to stay grounded as an art therapist as I work with Asian clients, including Aiko, who is a Japanese client of mine. Aiko came to see me for anxiety management. She calls me Sensei. She moved to the United States a couple of months ago because of her husband's job, and they would most likely go back to Japan in 2–3 years. This is her second time to stay in the United States. She worries about the environmental issues and climate changes, and her anxiety spikes when she sees the news about these topics. She spends countless hours on the Internet, searching for ways to remedy environmental damages caused by humans. In one of the sessions, I have suggested her to draw a container for her anxious thoughts. She engaged easily in guided imagery and came up with a Mason jar as a container (Figure 10.3). After she drew a jar with crayons, I asked her how her anxious thoughts would look like if she were to draw it. She created an image that looks like slime in purple-black color. "It is like an amoeba, and it's sticky." We talked about how she could use the Mason jar to seal the amoeba-like substances. She agreed to try it when an anxious thought came on to her next time. She'd imagine thought as an amoeba-like substance, and she'd put it in the jar and seal it.

In the subsequent session, I checked in with her about this strategy. She explained that it worked to a certain extent, but she did not use it much because she did not want to "see" the anxious thoughts she put in the jar previously. She then reported that imagery and drawing might not be as concrete enough for her to use as a strategy. As I acknowledged her findings, I shifted my session focus from art therapy to talk therapy with cognitive-behavioral therapy (CBT).

As I worked with her for two more sessions, I used talk therapy with CBT as a modality. I found myself feeling afraid to bring in art therapy directives back into her sessions. What was this fear about? I worried she might reject my idea, saying that art therapy is either childish or too abstract. The creative process in art therapy is not something that I can explain step-by-step in terms of how it works. You have to trust the process and allow the creative process to unfold. After all, I have seen so many transformations in clients through art therapy in the past 15 years of my practice. Why do I feel afraid to bring it to her? Last month, I just had another client who resisted collage making. He said it was too childish. I had no hesitation in bringing another task, mandala drawing, the week after to this client. Then I came to realize that I was trying to protect the image of me as the perfect, all-knowing, authority figure that

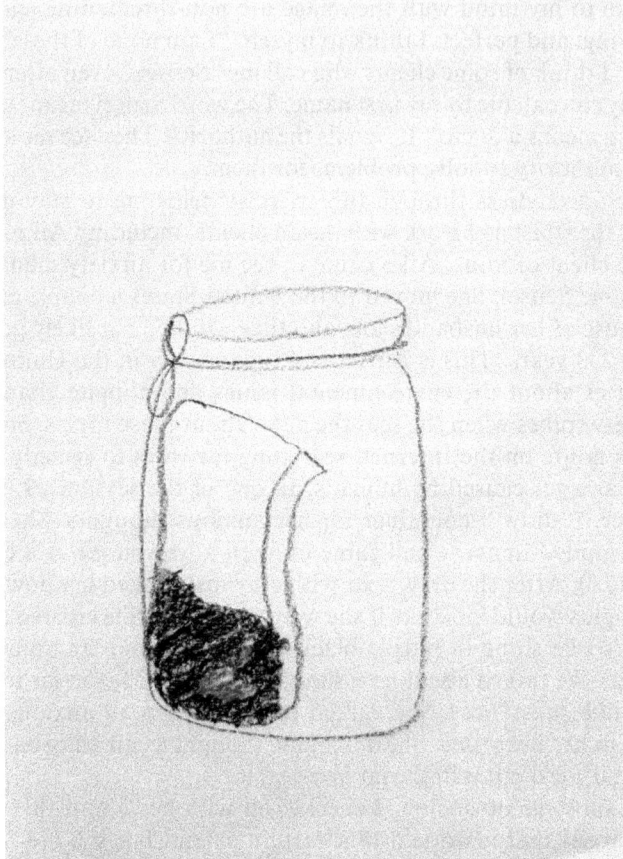

Figure 10.3 Drawing of Anxiety in a Container by a client.

I projected she needed, the figure I drew in the second self-exploration exercise. I was afraid of making a mistake and breaking the image of the all-knowing therapist. I also felt responsible for being an effective helper. It felt like a risk to bring in something that was not explainable word-by-word like art therapy. My realization of fear intrigued me. Was my assumption preventing Aiko to get what she needs in sessions? How did I presume if she would not benefit from art therapy?

In the session with Aiko after I gained this realization, I decided to experiment. I decided that I am going to engage her into an art therapy directive one more time and see how she would react. I needed to test if my own assumption about how I should be as her therapist in this intracultural encounter was clouding my clinical vision. In the next session, she came in with increased anxiety. She said she was captured by anxiety because of a particular article she read online about the environmental

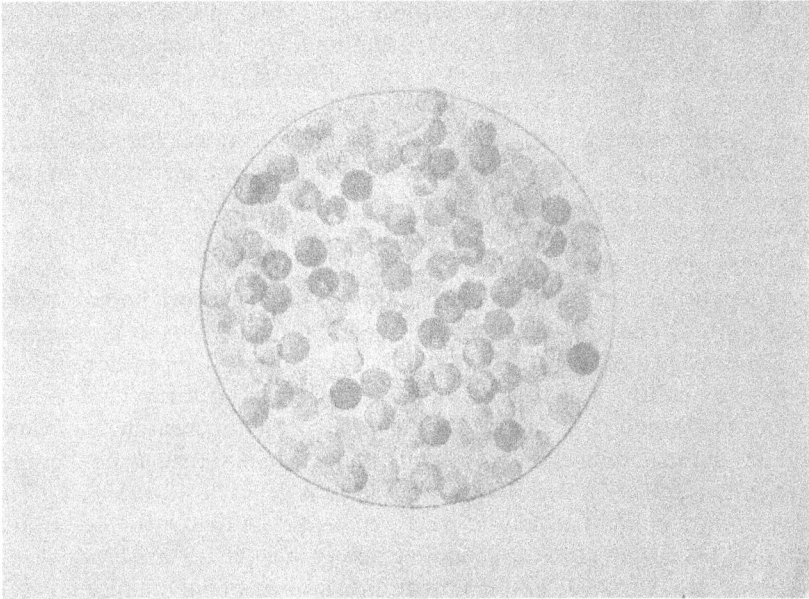

Figure 10.4 Dot Mandala by a client.

concern. She lost some sleep for the last several days. I introduced her mandala with the dotting technique, using the Dot Method (Lynch & Miller, 2016). I asked her to use the eraser on the pencil and stamp pad to make dot marks in a 4-inch circle drawn on a piece of paper until it was filled (Figure 10.4). After 10 minutes of dotting in silence, I asked Aiko how she felt. "I feel calmer," she replied. "It's like my mind is not thinking of anything. I see that it's good to just 'do' things." After she thanked me and left, I confirmed with myself that it was my projection of the all-knowing therapist that prevented me from using art therapy with Aiko before. I wanted her to see me as "Japanese enough" so that she felt she could relate to me. And unconsciously, I was trying to accomplish this by protecting the image of the all-knowing therapist.

Navigating Two Cultures

Bicultural competency can be a helpful concept as Asian art therapists manage the complexity of intracultural encounters. According to LaFromboise et al. (1993), individuals would need competency in the following elements so that they can effectively manage the process of living in two cultures: (a) knowledge of cultural beliefs and values, (b) positive attitudes toward both majority and minority groups, (c) bicultural efficacy ("the belief, or confidence, that one can live effectively, and in a satisfying manner, within two groups without compromising one's sense of cultural identity" (p. 404), (d) communication ability (verbally and non-verbally), (e) role repertoire (knowledge over situationally or culturally appropriate behaviors and roles), and (f) a sense of being grounded (i.e., having a well-developed support system in both cultures). LaFromboise et al. (1993) believed the alteration model of biculturalism was the most effective model. This model envisions that individuals can participate in two cultures successfully by altering their behaviors in each social context. LaFromboise et al. (1993) suggested that individuals can work on the aforementioned elements to achieve bicultural competency. Their concept can be helpful for Asian art therapists as a framework for becoming a bi-culturally competent therapist in a predominantly White profession.

Knowledge of cultural beliefs and values mentioned above can include how one's culture perceives art and what types of art are valued. As an Asian art therapist, it can be helpful to increase the awareness of how the art of racial minorities is typically non-existent in formal art therapy education. In the United States, what is considered as a "quality art" is determined by White, middle, and upper-class individuals who curate artworks and who have the economic power to value certain types of art as good art (Lippard, 1990). This pre-set notion of the quality creates racial inequality, making minorities' art perceived as not high quality and creating an assumption that they "just haven't got it yet (Lippard, 1990, p. 7)." It is only natural to think that what is valued in society is what is taught in colleges and universities. In formal education, art therapists would have a minimal exposure to build studio skills in arts often employed by minorities and their cultures for this reason. In addition, there are limited opportunities to expose them to challenge their Eurocentric perceptions of art in formal educational settings. The oil painting class is available, but not the Sumie painting class. Ceramics class is offered, but not the textile art class. If the formal art therapy education removed Asian art therapists too far from Asian forms of art to the point where we feel out of touch, it calls for an action to explore ways to enculture ourselves. Enculturation here refers to the process of integrating our own traditional culture back into the Westernized professional self.

In my experience, Asian clients would expect Asian art therapists like myself to know more about forms of art familiar in Asian communities than what our formal education provides. A Singaporean client of mine told me several months ago that she wanted to learn Kintsugi with my help. "I thought you would be a good teacher to do this since you are Japanese." Another client wanted to learn how to draw Manga comics. I have taken these situations as an opportunity to "enculturate" myself to Asian forms of art in an attempt to balance the personal and professional selves within me. And my own learning on Asian art forms has expanded my ability to see myself as a whole self in addition to accommodating my Asian clients' preferred ways to express and relate. In this enculturating endeavor, I have tried what I have never tried in my life: Kumihimo

(Braid making), Sumi-nagashi (marbling), printmaking, sumi-e (black ink painting), Omamori (amulet) making, and Origami.

There are many ways to work on achieving bicultural competency articulated by LaFrombise et al. (1993). Each Asian art therapist's effort to be bi-culturally competent with Asian and the dominant cultures would look different. Increasing knowledge over Asian forms of art is one method. Another method is to engage with other Asian therapists to create a supportive network. Acquiring additional counseling-related vocabulary in the Asian language also contributes to the integration of two cultures and bicultural competency. As an Asian art therapist continues to work on navigating two cultures, these methods and their self-awareness may support them by filling the gaps between what the formal education brought to them and what they encounter in intracultural relationships.

Conclusion

This chapter examined aspects to be considered in intracultural communication between Asian art therapists and Asian clients. Self-reflection to raise one's awareness of the relationship between the personal (Asian) self and the professional (Western-educated) self is recommended in order to practice culturally competent art therapy in intracultural encounters. It is also important to observe the difference in acculturation orientations between the therapist and the client and diversity within Asian as a race. As the Western art therapy education may not adequately prepare Asian art therapists to serve the needs of Asian clients, it is recommended that Asian art therapists invest efforts into striving for bicultural competency. This chapter was not written to stereotype Asian art therapists or Asian clients. The intention was to share my experience to validate the similar experiences of other Asian art therapists. I believe my experience of being an Asian in a predominantly White profession is more common than it has been written. Although this chapter included some recommendations, they do not apply to all Asian art therapists. In sharing her own personal and professional journey as an art therapist, Kaimal (2015) pointed out that it is important to seek out multiple storylines instead of stereotyping. This chapter should be considered as one of the multiple storylines that exist in the art therapy community.

References

American Art Therapy Association. (2011). Art therapy multicultural diversity competencies. Retrieved from https://arttherapy.org/wp-content/uploads/2017/06/Multicultural Competencies.pdf

Berry, J. W. (1980). Acculturation as varieties of adaptation. In A. M. Padilla (Ed.), *Acculturation, theory, models, and some new findings* (AAAS Selected Symposium, vol. 39, pp. 9–216). Westview Press.

Cabral, R. R. & Smith, T. B. (2011). Racial/ethnic matching of clients and therapists in mental health services: a meta-analytic review of preferences, perceptions, and outcomes. *Journal of Counseling Psychology, 58*(4), 537–54. doi: 10.1037/a0025266

Chang, D. F., & Yoon, P. (2011). Ethnic minority clients' perceptions of the significance of race in cross-racial therapy relationships. *Psychotherapy Research, 21*(5), 567–582. doi: 10.1080/10503307.2011.592549

De Vaus, J., Hornsey, M. J., Kuppens, P., & Bastian, B. (2018). Exploring the East-West divide in prevalence of affective disorder: A case for cultural differences in coping with negative emotion. *Personality and Social Psychology Review*, 22(3), 285–304.

Elkins, D. E., & Deaver, S. P. (2013). American art therapy association, Inc: 2013 membership survey report. *Art Therapy, 32*(2), 60–69. doi: 10.1080/07421656.2015.1028313

Fiorentine, R., & Hillhouse, M. P. (1999). Drug treatment effectiveness and client-counselor empathy. *Journal of Drug Issues, 29*, 59–74.

Flaskerud, J. H., & Liu, P. Y. (1991). Effects of an Asian client-therapist language, ethnicity and gender match on utilization and outcome of therapy. *Community Mental Health Journal, 27,* 31–42. doi: 10.1007/BF00752713

Ford, B. Q., Dmitrieva, J. O., Heller, D., Chentsova-Dutton, Y., Grossmann, I., Tamir, M., Mauss, I. B. (2015). Culture shapes whether the pursuit of happiness predicts higher or lower well-being. *Journal of Experimental Psychology General, 144*(6), 1053–1062.

Fors, M. (2018). *A grammar of power in psychotherapy: Exploring the dynamics of privilege*. Washington, DC: American Psychological Association. doi: 10.1037/0000086-000

Gamst, G., Dana, R. H., Der-Karabetian, A., & Kramer, T. (2004). Ethnic match and treatment outcomes for child and adolescent mental health center clients. *Journal of Counseling & Development, 82*, 457–465.

Gibson M. A. (2001). Immigrant adaptation and patterns of acculturation. *Human Development, 44*, 19–23. doi: 10.1159/000057037

Hocoy, D. (2002). Cross-cultural issues in art therapy. *Art Therapy, 19*(4), 141–145. doi:10.1080/07421656.2002.10129683

Kaimal, G. (2015). Evolving identities: The person(al), the profession(al), and the artist(ic), *Art Therapy, 32*(3), 136–141. doi: 10.1080/07421656.2015.1060840

Kim, B. S. K., Atkinson, D. R., & Yang, P. H. (1999). The Asian values scale: Development, factor analysis, validation, and reliability. *Journal of Counseling Psychology, 46*(3), 342–352. doi: 10.1037/0022-0167.46.3.342

Kim, B. S. K., & Omizo, M. M. (2005). Asian and European American cultural values, collective self-esteem, acculturative stress, cognitive flexibility, and general self-efficacy among Asian American college students. *Journal of Counseling Psychology, 52*(3), 412–419. doi: 10.1037/0022-0167.52.3.412

Kim-Goh, M., Choi, H., & Yoon, M. S. (2015). Culturally responsive counseling for Asian Americans: Clinician perspectives. *International Journal for the Advancement of Counselling, 37*, 63–76.

Kim, B. S., & Park, Y. S. (2015). Communication styles, cultural values, and counseling effectiveness with Asian Americans. *Journal of Counseling & Development, 93*(3), 269–279.

King, R. (2018). *Mindful of race: Transforming racism from the inside out*. Sounds True.

LaFromboise, T., Coleman, H. L. K., & Gerton, J. (1993). Psychological impact of biculturalism: Evidence and theory. *Psychological Bulletin, 114*(3), 395–412. doi: 10.1037/0033-2909.114.3.395

Li, L. C., & Kim, B.S. K. (2004). Effects of counseling style and client adherence to Asian values on counseling process with Asian American college students. *Journal of Counseling Psychology, 51*, 158–187. doi: 10.1037/00220167.51.2.158

Lippard, L. R. (1990). *Mixed blessings: New art in a multicultural America.* Pantheon Books.

Lynch, J., & Miller, A. (2016, July 9). The Dot Method for anxiety reduction [conference session]. The American Art Therapy Association's 47th Annual Conference. American Art Therapy Association, Baltimore, MD.

Meyer, O., Zane, N., & Cho, Y. I. (2011). Understanding the psychological processes of the racial match effect in Asian Americans. *Journal of Counseling Psychology, 58*(3), 335–345. doi: 10.1037/a0023605

Nipponda, Y. (2012). Japanese culture and therapeutic relationship. *Psychology and Culture, 10*(3). doi: 10.9707/2307-0919.1094

Shulman, L. (2015). *The skills of helping individuals, families, groups, and communities* (8th ed.). Cengage Learning.

Substance Abuse and Mental Health Services Administration. (2014). *Improving cultural competence: Treatment improvement protocol (TIP) series no. 59.* Rockville, MD: Substance Abuse and Mental Health Services Administration.

Sue, D. W., & Sue, D. (2003). *Counseling the culturally diverse: Theory and practice* (4th ed.). John Wiley & Sons, Inc.

Takeuchi, D. T., Sue, S., & Yeh, M. (1995). Return rates and outcomes from ethnicity-specific mental health programs in Los Angeles. *American Journal of Public Health, 85*, 638–643. doi: 10.2105/AJPH.85.5.638

U.S. Census Bureau. (2000). America's Asian population Demographic Patterns & Trends. Retrieved from: http://proximityone.com/asian_demographics.htm

Utsey, S. O., Gernat, C. A., & Hammar, L. (2005). Examining White counselor trainees' reactions to racial issues in counseling and supervision dyads. *Counseling Psychologist, 33*(4), 449–478. doi: 10.1177/0011000004269058

VandenBos, G. R. (Ed.). (2007). *APA dictionary of psychology.* American Psychological Association.

Vasquez, M. J. T. (2007). Cultural difference and the therapeutic alliance: An evidence-based analysis. *American Psychologist, 62*(8), 878–885. doi: 10.1037/0003-066X.62.8.878

Wong, E. C., Beutler, L. E., & Zane, N. W. (2007). Using mediators and moderators to test assumptions underlying culturally sensitive therapies: An exploratory example. *Cultural Diversity and Ethnic Minority Psychology, 13*(2), 169–177. doi: 10.1037/1099-9809.13.2.169

Wu, I. H., & Windle, C. (1980). Ethnic specificity in the relative minority use and staffing of community mental health centers. *Community Mental Health Journal, 16,* 156–168. doi: 10.1007/BF00778587

11 Possible Use of Art-Based Supervision in Japan

Reiko Fujisawa

Introduction

I was born and raised in Japan. I was already an adult when I moved to New York (NY). I've been practicing art therapy for nearly 20 years after receiving a master's degree from New York University. I worked at public and private hospitals in New York City (NYC), mainly for inpatient psychiatric patients with children, adults, and older adults. Currently, I am a child psychology specialist at the Japanese government and provide counseling in Tokyo for adolescents and adults. During my art therapy practice in the United States, receiving supervision was an essential part of my professional life. It was a secure home base where I stored energy, increased motivation, and received inspiration and encouragement. I cannot imagine how I survived my career in NYC without supervision. After 15 years of practice in the United States, I returned to Japan. To my surprise, I learned many professionals do not have supervision after completing master's degrees. Some told me that they do not have positive impressions with supervision experiences. I became interested in looking into this trend in Japan. Psychology Professional School Five Academy (2018) in Japan defines supervision as "professional guidance from a supervisor who has the rich clinical experience to a supervisee who is less experienced, and the guidance includes educational, administrative, and supportive functions" (p. 342). I believe in having more two-way relationships and the vital alliance between a supervisor and a supervisee. They learn about each other having a compassionate, safe place to discuss clinical cases and ethics and helping supervisees professionally grow with self-confidence (Creaner, 2013).

Mental Health Field in Japan

Before discussing clinical supervision in Japan, I think it is necessary to inform you about the Japanese mental health system to provide a better view of supervisions. Traditionally speaking, Japanese people are hesitant to talk about their behavioral or psychological problems with someone outside of their family members. It is considered shameful and stigmatized to visit a therapist. Because of these cultural values and a denial of the service demand, Japan had obstacles expanding and accepting the need for mental health practices. There was no known system of having licensed psychologists in Japan until recently. In 2018, the first licensed profession in psychology was created, and it is called "Certified Public Psychologist." This can be a deceitful license, and I will refer to this license later.

In Japan, students who graduated from a master's degree in clinical psychology programs do not pursue doctors' degrees unless they wish to be an academic professor or a researcher. According to the Japanese Society of Certified Clinical Psychologists (2020), career opportunities of master's level professionals vary, in educational, medical & public health settings, welfare, legal and probation settings, vocations, academic institutions, and private practices. To practice psychotherapy, they must be board certified. Although the Japanese Society of Certified Clinical Psychologists has more than 30 years of history, the certification process has never received regulated licensures by the government. Instead, board-certified psychotherapists are encouraged to obtain the above-mentioned "Certified Public Psychologist." This is an only national license given to those who are specialized in counseling or psychotherapy. Many positions in mental health settings require employees to have this license so that psychiatrists can prescribe treatments such as psychological testing by clinical psychologists. These services can be billed through health insurance.

The certified public psychologist is an acquired trend in Japanese society. Doctor's level psychologists and people with only a high school diploma with five years of on-site experiences in mental health settings can apply for the license. Luckily, the stricter law will regulate this from 2022, that applicants must hold at least a bachelor's degree. From the year 2018 to 2022, anyone can apply for the credential regardless of one's educational backgrounds, as long as one has worked in the fields of a public health system, educational settings, legal/criminal systems, and vocational/labor settings for more than five years. So, nurses at hospitals and probation officers at family courts can receive the credential.

The use of professional titles, such as psychologists or psychotherapists, is subdued and ambiguous in Japan. This reflects how little they acknowledge the field of mental health. In the United States, one must hold a doctor's degree to be called a psychologist. However, in Japan, the psychologist's job title becomes even murkier when translated from Japanese to English. There are two recognized psychologists' job titles: (1) 臨床心理士, Rinsho (clinical) Shinri-Shi (psychology worker), and (2) 公認心理士, Konin (certified) Shinri-Shi (psychology worker). When

Japanese psychologists explain their job titles in English, they unknowingly say they are clinical psychologists but without doctor's degrees.

The work responsibilities of clinical psychologists and certified public psychologists are overlapped for the most part, but clinical psychologists are expected to provide psychotherapy or counseling. They are also encouraged to research to improve their professional skills and to report continuing education credits when they renew their certifications every five years. Certified public psychologists, on the other hand, are not required to do so. Once you obtain the license, it will be permanent unless you violate laws.

Further, the field of Japanese social work also experiences slow-moving development. This is a much-needed profession, especially in child welfare agencies, nursing homes, and hospital settings. There are three kinds of national licenses in social work; certified social worker, psychiatric social worker, and certified care worker. The educational requirement is generally a bachelor's degree, or one can apply for this license if he/she completes a specific vocational school program. There is yet another way to function as a social worker. When a person is employed as a municipal worker and being told to take a position at one of the Child Protective Services, he or she acts as a welfare social worker receiving the immediate job training at the site. Only 40% of child welfare workers are legitimate, government-certified social workers, but the rest became social workers by chance (Okubo, 2019).

It is not illegal for persons to identify themselves as therapists without proper educations in Japan, and some are very successful. They not only provide "therapy" to the public but also published numerous books and are welcomed expertise on media alongside more scientific scholars. Some uneducated therapists built professional schools to teach their unique techniques and to produce the next generation of poorly trained therapists. It is possible to harm clients more without having any intent. However, ordinary Japanese citizens are attracted to the therapists who talk about captivating topics on media without a grain of salt. It is not common for them to seek help from licensed professionals. They tend to look for instant solutions and immediate gratifications. They are unfamiliar with the idea of maintaining regular therapy sessions, which are common in the United States. Exploring one's inner world means that a person has to face his/her deep-seated issues that Japanese people tend to ignore. Instead, they prefer brief and direct advice and to look for counselors who can provide straightforward steps on what to do or what not to do as in coaching. Besides, Japanese health insurance does not cover private therapy fees. Only licensed professionals, whom I previously mentioned, could be billed to health insurance. Continuing to see a private psychotherapist is simply not an option for many.

Supervision in Japan

There are Japanese mental health supervisors with superb experiences and skills. But they are hard to find. Indeed, what I tell you here does not apply to everything that happens in Japan. When I returned in 2016, I discovered that mental health workers had unsupportive supervision, and most of them did not attend regular supervision after graduation. Clinicians, who continue supervision voluntarily, are the minority. As I mentioned in the beginning, my experiences of supervision in the United States were positive and satisfying. It was heartbreaking to hear about my colleagues' supervision experiences that were hurtful and unsafe. Some of them became tearful while they were sharing the stories.

I discuss some possible causes of these negative experiences based on reports from my colleagues:

1 The system of clinical and supportive supervision is not established.
2 Clinicians' past, repeated experiences of unsupportive supervision.
3 Lack of fund to seek supervision.
4 Lack of resources to find supervisors.
5 A misconception that supervision is for beginners.

Commonly, the students are not well informed about the importance of supervision during their studies. Supervisors themselves are not sure about the significance. According to my colleagues, students feel that some supervisors are abusive by making students feel ashamed of their works. It creates an anxiety-provoking and stressful environment. In addition, the average salary of clinical psychologists makes it impossible to pay supervision fees at the beginning of their careers. They might also think that having a supervisor makes them appear incompetent because of their belief that they are for beginners as well as a sign of weakness to seek help for themselves.

On the other hand, Japanese social workers have increased their awareness and the importance of clinical and supportive supervision. Japanese child protection services are criticized for the insufficiency to assist and to protect children's lives. Thus, there are many cases of children's death caused by caregivers every year. What they are trying to do is to establish a firm foundation of supervision so that they can provide better support for children and families (Kuraishi, 1996; Shiota, 2013; Kanbayashi, 2017). Tsushima (2000) stated that she thought she had to be omnipotent always to make the right decision as a supervisor; this adds to the misconception of supervision. Shiota (2013) pointed out that supervision at welfare settings means, help, or guidance provided by people who have worked longer at the site but are not necessarily specialized in the field of mental health. These patchwork supervisors seem to ignore the supervisees' profession and to prevent them from improving their professional skills. Shiota (2013) continued saying that administrative supervision is readily available in many settings, but they do not help the growth of supervisees. Ishida (2000) stated that supervisors often scold supervisees for insufficient supervision by blaming supervisees for their incompetency, personalities, or even upbringings. It is now clear that in these circumstances, supervisees lose motivation to seek supervisors (Ueda, 1999).

Art Therapy in Japan

As I aforementioned, the field of Japanese mental health is underdeveloped, and art therapy is no exception. Seki (2016), an art therapist trained in the United States, said that it is becoming more common to hear the term art therapy in Japan. However, it is still not widely recognized. Currently, there are no bachelor's or master's programs in art therapy. Some universities offer art therapy courses, and students can choose to take it as an elective. But these courses are not customary in most of the Japanese universities. Since 2019, one art therapy pilot program has started at Tsukuba University with US funding. Mrs. Karen Pence, the wife of the US vice president, is a big supporter of this program. If this goes well, it may continue as a regular course. It is not sure if the course will offer a degree, though. Many private vocational schools provide art therapy instructions, but people who do not have a proper art therapy education run these schools. They studied sociology, psychology, or even economics. Many faculties of these schools are graduates from the same schools. The teaching varies from the techniques of self-care to real therapy interventions. These programs are useful for students who already have mental health backgrounds and can utilize art therapy as their new modalities.

One of these vocational art therapy schools is called Quest Art Therapy & Training Analysis and affiliated to the Canadian International Institute of Art Therapy (CiiAT). They have the Japan International Program of Art Therapy in Tokyo (JIPATT). Faculties that are all trained in art therapy in Northern America, including me, constitute it. This is the only art therapy program in Japan to offer both art therapy and supervision. After completion, students will receive clinical art therapy diplomas from CiiAT.

In the JIPATT, students must complete 350 hours of internship, 30 group supervision, and five individual ones. Internship sites include: after school programs, vocational assistance programs, nursing homes, a group home for severely disabled individuals, to mention a few. Some sites do not practice having clinical charts. Even when they are available, they are often out of students' reach. Clients' sensitive information is verbally handed down to the students who have no opportunities to attend clinical or treatment plan meetings. Besides, they hardly have chances to learn how DSM-5 diagnoses manifest on a client because it is not used to discuss clients' psychiatric symptoms. The students provide monthly, or at most, bi-weekly group therapy and inform the team about what was happening in groups. Worse, they do not have site supervisors, not to mention art therapy but also for general concerns or emergencies. Staff members and clients also show blunt skepticism due to a lack of understanding and wonder whether students offer art therapy or recreational activities. These circumstances are not born out of dysfunctional internship programs or the abilities of students. It is merely Japan's inadequate infrastructure in the field of mental health.

Art Therapy Supervision

I have been an off-site supervisor for approximately two years at JIPATT. All students are part-time students and have non-art therapy careers. My goals are to provide supportive space and to give positive, frank feedback. During the hour of supervision, I am impressed by the students' enthusiasm to gain a better insight into clients' artwork and the art-making process despite challenging situations. Mostly, I offer verbal supervision, but one day, I gave a try to art-based supervision. The art-based supervision consists of me giving students a directive to make images of their countertransference. Despite the direct and challenging theme, they were receptive. I also felt a rapport with the students trusting that we could create a safe environment to focus on the process. Kitazoe (2005) emphasized that reviewing how to conduct supervision by both a supervisor and a supervisee, and discussing the purposes of supervision, is a step to improve the quality of supervision. Due to the COVID-19 pandemic, following supervision examples were conducted on-line.

Student A's internship site was an employment support center. Based on my directive, she created an image of her client, who was unemployed and diagnosed with a developmental disorder. She felt challenging to relate to him and felt scared of him. She had no clue what he was thinking and felt as if he blamed her for no particular reasons. There seemed to be a veil between them, and she acknowledged a feeling of superficiality when she interacts with him during art therapy sessions. She drew the image of the client twice. On her first drawing (not pictured), the client's feature had some cracks. She explained that the client in her artwork was about to break; she became uncomfortable with the image. Then she quickly rationalized to say that their therapeutic relationship was not that bad after all. So, she tore the work and created Figure 11.1. After making the second one, she said she could take a slight distance away from this client even though there is still a veil in the image. This helped

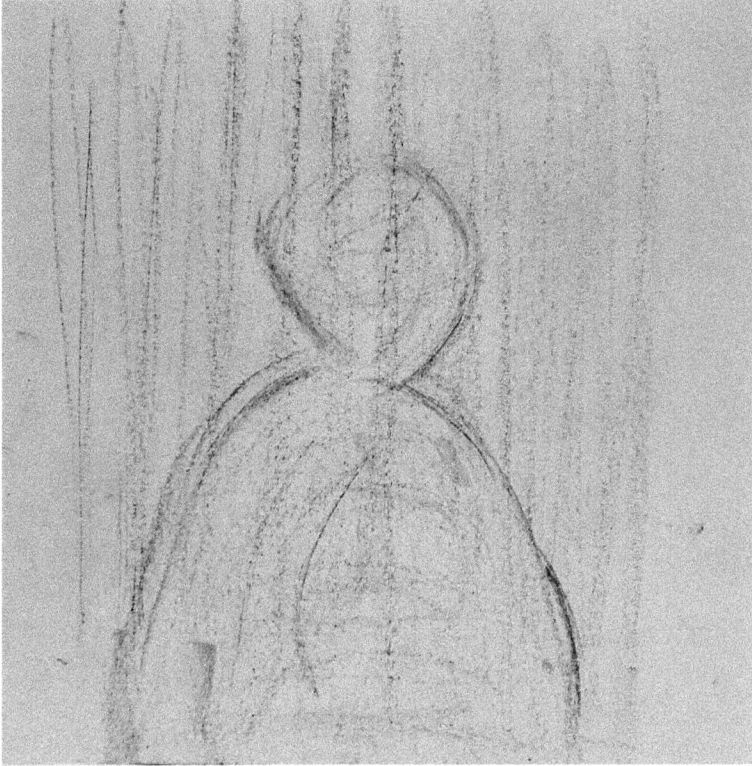

Figure 11.1 What Provokes My Anxiety. Drawing by a supervisee.

her see the situation objectively, and she looked forward to having a session with a newfound self-confidence.

It was only Student B's second supervision session while she told me that the issue of countertransference has never occurred to her. She just said she knew the word. Her internship site was at a nursing home and created an image of a client who was always irritable (Figure 11.2). She said, "This is well done. This looks just like her." She also described that the client was rough as jagged rocks. The client complained about everything, including art therapy, except when student B brought materials such as tiddlywinks and artificial flowers. Seeing the client smile made the student think, "I do not really dislike her." I asked the student why she thought of it, and she took the time to explain. I helped her to explore her feelings, and the student said she felt being unacknowledged and devalued by this client as a therapist. Student B then related this feeling of being an art teacher at an elementary school where she does not receive enough appreciation.

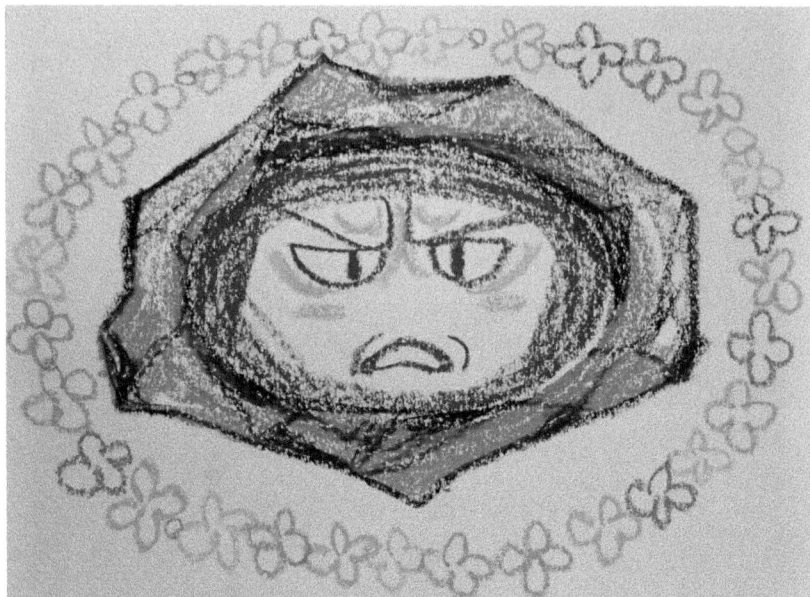

Figure 11.2 Untitled. Drawing by a supervisee.

In the previous supervision with student C, I suggested practicing clear professional boundaries with a client, a boy, who was diagnosed with ADHD because she was increasingly emotionally invested in him. Student C's internship site was an afterschool program for children with developmental disorders. She was letting the boy take over the helm of the therapy session and was unable to objectively analyze the situation why the session became out of control. After my advice, she was back in charge of leading the session again by giving him the freedom to enjoy his art-making process and tasks while maintaining her professional grounding. By creating even, emotional tension between them, her interaction with the child significantly changed. She made a sculpture (Figure 11.3) representing her ability to safely share the transitional space with him (Winnicott, 1971). A small circle with a post represented student C, connected to another small circle (the boy). The two circles look as if they are throwing a tiny yarn ball playfully that represented her distanced attention to the boy. Student C terminated therapy with him without being overly emotional. She realized creating this sculpture and reviewing it in our supervision session made her experience more meaningful.

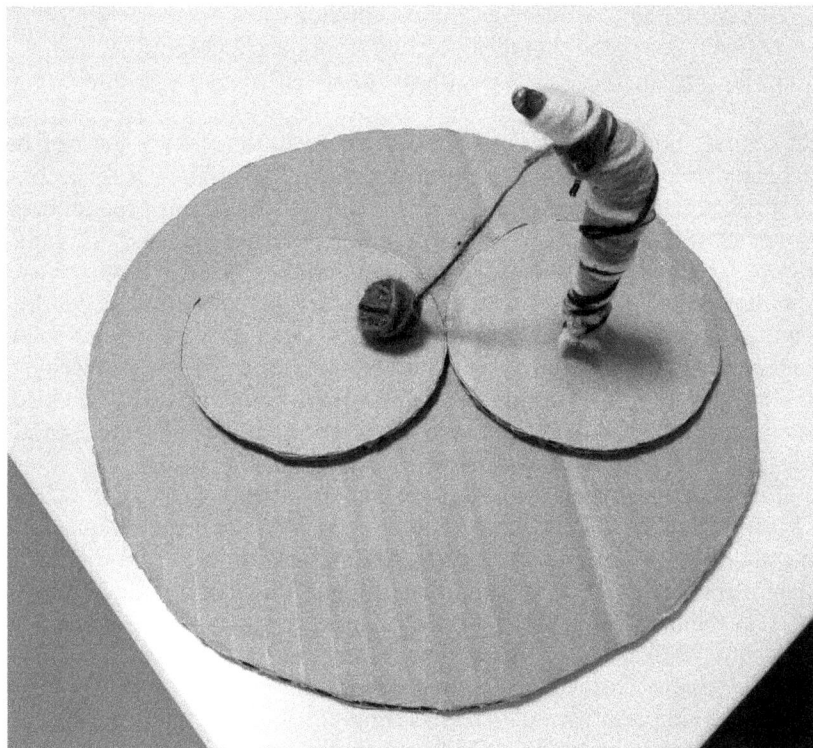

Figure 11.3 Untitled. Drawing by a supervisee.

Conclusion

Japanese mental health supervisors and professionals should provide a more supportive and nurturing environment for supervisees to develop their clinical skills. Post-session art-makings, not only by art therapists but also by other mental health professionals, can be integrated into supervision. The creative process may help supervisees to feel less anxious while promoting a better alliance with each other. It also allows supervisees to separate their subjective emotions and experiences and to make physical distance visible, increasing self-awareness (Deaver & McAuliffe, 2009; Guiffrida et al., 2007; Harter, 2007; Jackson et al., 2008). Making invisible visible in the art may help supervisee not to take their experiences with their clients too personally. Ishiyama (1988) also suggested that the emphasis on visually oriented process promotes effective and engaging communication to understand clinical cases better. According to Keilo's study (1991, as cited in Deaver & Shiflett, 2011), there are five functions of post-session art-making, and it helps:

Developing empathy with the client.
Clarifying the therapist's feelings.

Exploring the preconscious and unconscious.
Differentiating the therapist's feeling from the client's and
Exploring the therapeutic relationship. (p. 263).

Of course, non-art therapy supervisees' resistance making art can be expected because most of them have not used art materials for a long time. A supervisor then must stress the quality of the end product does not matter, but the process of art-making matters. Processing the experience together in a safe environment is crucial. Also, the supervisor should be flexible, whether to make art during supervision or beforehand. Stephanie L. Harter (2007), an American clinical psychologist, reflected her personal growth through art-making. She acknowledged the art process as a "deeply personal way of knowing" (p. 177). Also, Wadeson (2003) wrote, "art offers us for reflection, insight, understanding, and problem solving around work with clients" (p. 208).

To change the current situations in Japanese supervision and the field of mental health, the government needs to make room for a few improvements. First, they need to acknowledge that there are separate entities in the mental health workers by making uniquely customized guidelines to protect them and the public. Second, higher education degrees need to be almost obligatory in each profession instead of the length of employment by poorly trained staff. Lastly, continuing financial and economic support from the government to accommodate high-quality training systems and resources. They might be the windows to the increased awareness of citizens' mental health issues, and therapists' life-long learning process that advocates for supervision are not only for inexperienced professionals. These things won't happen overnight. But I believe the art-based supervision can create a safe environment for supervisors and supervisees of all levels to discuss their real and authentic experiences with their clients.

References

Creaner, M. (2013). *Getting the best out of supervision in counseling & psychotherapy: A guide for the supervisee*. Sage Publications Ltd.

Deaver, S. P., & McAuliffe, G. (2009). Reflective visual journaling during art therapy and counseling internships: A qualitative study. *Reflective Practice*, *10*(5), 615–632. https://doi.org/10.1080/14623940903290687

Deaver, S. P., & Shiflett, C. (2011) Art-based supervision techniques. *The Clinical Supervisor*, *30*(2), 257–276. http://doi.org/10.1080/07325223.2011.619456

Guiffrida, D. A., Jordan, R., Saiz, S., & Barnes, K. L. (2007). The use of metaphor in clinical supervision. *Journal of Counseling & Development*, *85*(4), 393–400. https://doi.org/10.1002/j.1556-6678.2007.tb00607.x

Harter, S. (2007). Visual art making for therapist growth and self-care. *Journal of Constructivist Psychology*, *20*(2), 167–182. https://doi.org/10.1080/10720530601074721

Ishida, A. (2000). *Koukatekina su-pa-bijyon wo sasaeru yottuno jyouken: So-sharu wa-ku kenkyu [Four conditions of supporting effective supervision: Social work research]*. Aikawa Books.

Ishiyama, F. I. (1988). A model of visual case processing using metaphors and drawings. *Counselor Education and Supervision, 28*, 153–161. https://doi.org/10.1002/j.1556-6978.1988.tb01781.x

Jackson, S. A., Muro, J., Lee, Y. T., & DeOrnellas, K. (2008). The sacred circle: Using mandalas in counselor supervision. *Journal of Creativity in Mental Health, 3*(3), 201–211. https://doi.org/10.1080/15401380802369164

Japanese Society of Certified Clinical Psychologists (n.d.). Rinsho shinrisi no katudou no ba [Places where certified clinical psychologists have jobs]. Retrieved May 11, 2020, from http://www.jsccp.jp/person/scene.php

Kanbayashi, M. (2017). Su-pa-bijyon ni okeru Su-pa-baiza- ga motiiru sukiru: so-sharu wa-ka- ni yoru su-pa-bijyon no situteki chosa [Supervisor's skills on supervision session: Qualitative study of supervision by social worker]. *Nihon Fukushi University Shakai Fukushi gaku, 58*(1), 71–85. https://doi.org/10.24469/jssw.58.1_71

Kitazoe, N. (2005). Su-pa-bijyon, ke-su kanfarensu no kenkyu: Su-pa-baiji- heno anke-to yori [Study of supervision and case conference: From the questionnaire to supervisees]. *Naruto University of Education (Arts and Social Science) Kenkyu Kiyo, 20*, 23–30. https://id.ndl.go.jp/bib/7305554

Kuraishi, T. (1996). Gennnshokuin su-pa-bijyon no Igigenjyo oyobi kadai nituiteno kousatu (dai ni hokoku): Shakaifukushi shisetu deno su-pa-bijyon [A Study on the significance of the current staff supervision/current situation and issues (the second report): Development of supervision in social welfare facilities]. *Shakai Mondai Kenkyu, 45*(2), 143–161. http://doi.org/10/24729/00003427

Okubo, M. (2019, March 25). Hitodebusoku, towarerushitu jidoufukushishi ni hituyouna senmonsei toha? [Lack of manpower, questionable quality, and expertise required for child welfare workers?]. *Asahishinbun Digital*. https://www.asahi.com/articles/ASM3H5FMJM3HUTIL02F.html?iref=pc_ss_date

Seki, N. (2016). *Clinical art therapy: Theory and practice*. Nihon Hyoron Sha.

Psychology Professional School Five Academy [Shinrisennmongakkou Five Academy]. (2018). *Rinsho shinrishi shiken tekisuto to mondaishuu [Clinical psychologist exam: Text and workbook]*. (2018–2019 version). Natsume Sha.

Shiota, S. (2013, March). Su-pa-bijyon ga fukushi genba ni nedukanai riyu ni tsuiteno kosatsu [Consideration about why supervision does not take root in the welfare field]. *Hanazono University Social Welfare Gakubu Kenkyu Kiyo, 21*, 31–40. http://id.nii.ac.jp/1175/00000202/

Tsushima, S. (2000, June). Shakkai fukushi jissen niokeru su-pa-bijyon [Supervision on social welfare practice]. *Gendai no Esupuri, 395*, 73–82. https://id.ndl.go.jp/bib/5369162

Ueda, H. (1999). Shosharuwa-ku wo jissen suru soshiki no sennryakuteki kasseika: kanryososiki no doutaika [Strategic activation of organizations that practice social work: mobilization of bureaucratic organizations]. *Kougakukan University Shakai Fukushi Ronshu, 2*, 173–179. https://id.ndl.go.jp/bib/5454149

Wadeson, H. (2003). Making art for professional processing. *Art Therapy: Journal of the American Art Therapy Association, 20*(4), 208–218. https://doi.org/10.1080/07421656.2003.10129606

Winnicott, D. W. (1971). *Playing and reality*. Tavistock Publications Ltd.

Conclusion

A Need for Cognitive Diversity in Multicultural Training

Megu Kitazawa

I write this conclusion in April 2020, in a time when schools and stores across many parts of the globe are closed and we confine ourselves to our homes to avoid social contact. In supermarkets, toilet papers, flour, and baking yeast are flying off shelves faster than ever. Guidelines such as social distancing, keeping a minimum of two meters away from one another, self-quarantining for 14 days, and singing "Happy Birthday" twice while washing our hands dictate our new way of living. The field of art therapy has not been spared from the effects of the coronavirus pandemic. There have been more discussions about sanitizing art materials, using Zoom or Skype to conduct virtual art therapy sessions, and protecting ourselves by wearing masks and gloves. The challenges we now face include not only ethnically diversifying our field, but also increasing digital diversity to overcome the crisis and maintaining the highest standard of ethics. Many of our fellow art therapists are parents who, on top of preparing three meals a day, also homeschool their children while working from home.

Regrettably, two other authors I had lined up for this book have had to withdraw their contribution as other new and urgent commitments take priority in this unprecedented and demanding state of affairs. While I am discouraged by the loss of their chapters, I feel more disheartened that this year's Art Therapy conference in Washington DC, which looks promisingly different, may be canceled. As I browse through the conference program, I notice that one of the keynote speakers is Asian. Reading through the rest of the program, I'm also excited to find lineups for presentations by Japanese, South Korean, and Taiwanese art therapists, sessions about Chinese Calligraphy, and collage-making in Singapore. At the same time, there are programs titled, "White Privilege in Art Therapy," "White Feminist Accountability in Organizational Systems," and "Interrupting Racism through Confronting White Fragility," in recognition of the White privilege and culture that pervade the art therapy discipline. I'm also particularly thrilled to see the family-friendly environment conference organizers are creating in providing a lactation room for nursing mothers and organizing Halloween activities for young children. These were all unimaginable back when my children were newborns. I can't help but feel elated by such positive and encouraging news, especially during this crisis like this. It's a conference that will bring together people from all walks of life and validate our sense of self and inclusivity and I hope for things to improve sooner rather than later and that the conference can take place as scheduled.

The era of Edith Kramer in art therapy has long gone. Kramer believed that art therapists needed part-time jobs to brush up on their artistic skills during non-working hours (Acosta, 2018). Today, this would be impossible for most of us. In this modern era, it is almost standard to find art therapists working as social workers and psychologists, often with double or even triple credentials to survive and to protect what we love: art therapy. Meanwhile, the "American Dream" that my father's generation pursued does not seem to exist in the field. Regardless of whether we're Asian, art therapists face huge hurdles in being taken seriously and professionally in a field where credibility is measured by the number of research papers published and the grasp of the English language. Despite our credentials, some of us continue to face economic challenges such as low-paying salaries and having to rely on our partners for financial support in order to continue practicing. It's also common to require doctorate degrees from other disciplines such as psychology and social work to be able to get hired as an educator or even be considered "real" art therapists at conferences.

The new generation of art therapists faces the same challenges we did years prior: the lack of art therapy students from different ethnic backgrounds and the low recruitment rate of non-White professors (Awais & Yali, 2015). It is appalling how certain White art therapists believe we have achieved our goal in diversifying our profession and fail to see just how White-dominated the discipline continues to be (Awais & Yali, 2015). In my opinion, the lack of progress in this regard is apparent simply by browsing through past conference brochures. What are we missing? Is it the development of effective multicultural training programs or a higher recruitment of students from different ethnic backgrounds? Or is it as simple as preaching a sense of empathy with one another and giving chances to those who love art therapy instead of counting the number of credentialed alphabets that follow after one's name?

Compared to the excellent selection of Japanese food in NYC, the variety of gastronomy in Berlin can be a letdown. After much discussion with my Japanese friends, we arrived at the conclusion, "They just don't get it, do they?" I draw similarities between this and multicultural training in the field of art therapy in that we lack the understanding of what is missing, which hinders our ability to improve. What ingredients do we need to spice up multicultural training and make it less defensive and resistive so that we can use our five senses to enjoy learning and absorb the material? How can we, Asian art therapists, contribute when, more often than not, getting hired as an educator is almost unthinkable? This is especially pertinent for Asian art therapists who immigrated to the United States as adults and face language barriers (imperfect written and oral English skills), have distinct cultural mannerisms (not as verbally expressive or too timid), and lack the financial means to pursue further education (having already spent their family's money to enroll in an art therapy program in the United States).

My move to Germany was my second immigration and integration into White society. Once again, I found myself facing the same struggles I did in my move to the United States with a second encounter with language barriers and cultural differences. The ignorant hostility and misunderstandings I face in my everyday life is on a whole new level compared to the racial slurs I used to receive from my patients. Shopkeepers in the former East German territories can be outright rude when they see non-White people or English-speaking foreigners. Here, not only do I represent Japan, but I've also taken on another stereotype. I am also an "American."

The American accent is a common dinner conversation topic, in which people often mock the way the "R" sounds are pronounced and imitate accents. While I have no trouble rolling my tongue to pronounce the American "R," the German "R" proves impossible for me. I rationalize their behavior not as disrespect but a reflection of the German's straightforward and direct speech, free of any sugar-coating. Where an American might remark, "Did you cut your hair? You look great," a German would probably ask, "Why did you cut your hair?" They might also say, "This lasagna is very dry. What did you do?" instead of refraining from commenting.

Saying nothing is destructive in the field of art therapy. In our attempt to encourage cognitive diversity, there may just be something that we could take out of the Germans' communication playbook. Cognitive diversity refers to the different ways people processing complicated situations and sharing their knowledge, ideas, and opinions (Reynolds & Lewis, 2017). This definition may ring a bell and most may think they understand it, but misinterpretations are common. For example, a group of art therapists hailing from varying ethnic backgrounds, ages, and socio-economic statuses gathering to solve a problem represents cultural diversity in the field. But in spite of the wide range of backgrounds and the combined intellect and brilliance of these professionals, the problem will not be solved effectively. Having undergone the same education and training, they have the same approaches, ideas, perspectives, and views. The less homogenous their approaches, the more effective the process and the more successful the outcome; this varied approach emphasizes what we don't know, more than what we already know. We may know how to make lasagna, but we don't know why it turns out dry and thus don't know how to improve it. So let's strive to make as many different kinds of lasagna as we can.

I've been living in Berlin for nearly four years. To be frank, I'm now rather fond of the unpleasant shopkeepers. I've adopted an empathetic approach towards them, which has, in turn, drawn out their compassionate side. In my communication, I try not to be as defensive as native Berliners. But as humans, we all have inherent biases against others and we stick to what we know, which leads to "empathy deficit" (Miller, 2019). It's also a natural tendency to cluster among those with similar educational and racial backgrounds and socio-economic statuses. We, art therapists, often describe ourselves as naturally empathetic towards people in need. If this were true, we should expand our study into multiculturalism through the foundation of empathy on which Asian art therapists' unique experiences are based. It is my hope for this book to represent a first step towards reinventing empathetic multicultural training and towards each other.

References

Acosta, I. (2018). Teaching with Edith. In L. Gerity, & S. A. Anand (Eds.), *The legacy of Edith Kramer: A multifaceted view* (pp. 67–70). Routledge.

Awais, Y. J., & Yali, A. M. (2015). Efforts in increasing racial and ethnic diversity in the field of art therapy. *Art Therapy: Journal of the American Art Therapy Association, 32*:3, 112–119. https://doi.org/10.1080/07421656.2015.1060842

Miller, C. (2019). How to be more empathetic: A year of better living guide. *New York Times*. https://www.nytimes.com/guides/year-of-living-better/how-to-be-more-empathetic

Reynolds, A., & Lewis, D. (March 30, 2017). Teams solve problems faster when they're more cognitively diverse. *Harvard Business Publishing*. https://hbr.org/2017/03/teams-solve-problems-faster-when-theyre-more-cognitively-diverse

Index

AATA 1, 27, 88, 128; art therapist locator 88; conference 3, 77, 151, 152; membership 27; open forum 1
acculturation 14–15, 53, 123, 124, 126, 128, 129, 135
African-American 2, 4, 20, 26, 67, 76, 77, 78, 89
Americanized 2, 38, 49, 123
anxiety 18, 46, 63, 94, 98, 99, 122, 131, 132, 142, 145
art therapy: classes 4; student 2, 3, 4, 6, 18, 26, 30, 55, 76, 86, 94, 96, 127, 143, 144, 145, 146, 152
Asian art therapist 1, 3, 4, 5, 6, 25, 55, 76, 77, 83, 108, 121, 123, 124, 127, 128, 133, 134, 135, 153, 154
Asian-American(s) 4, 12, 41, 62, 86, 97, 108, 122, 123, 124
assimilation 15, 16, 25, 123, 128, 129
awareness 2, 3, 50, 51, 52, 53, 55, 56, 73, 105, 134, 135, see also self-awareness

bias(es) 20, 26, 38, 49, 50, 52, 68, 128, 154
bicultural: competencies 5–6, 133–135; identity 4, 134, see also identity
bindi 16, 17, 66, 67
black(s) 2, 18, 21, 30, 57, 67, 89
Bowen, M. 3
Brahmin 10, 11, 12, 19
Buddhist 4, 26, 41, 43, 48

caste 4, 10–11, 19, 66
casteism 10–11

Caucasian(s) 48, 51, 76, 90, 121
CBT 97, 131
China 2, 4, 26, 28, 29, 30, 31, 59, 60, 61, 62, 63, 89
cognitive diversity 151, 153
color blind 4, 25, 29, 30
countertransference 9, 22, 29, 63, 128, 144, 145
cross-cultural 41, 44, 47, 48, 50, 53, 54
cultural competence 3, 51, 65,
cultural diversity, see also diversity
cultural humility 5, 48, 51, 65, 68, 73
cultural identity 4, 14, 41, 51, 59, 60, 65, 87, 90, 128, 129, 133–4, see also identity
culturally humble 66, 74, 120

depression 5, 52, 96, 97, 98, 99, 101, 102, 104, 108, 111, 122
discrimination 4, 10, 18, 19, 50, 55, 56, 129
diversity 4, 5, 18, 50, 52, 77, 88, 121, 129, 135, 151, 153; cultural 26, 46, 77, 79, 86, 87, 107, 153; workshop 21
drawing(s) 31, 34, 36, 45, 57, 58, 59, 69, 70, 71, 72, 83, 84, 87, 99, 101, 102, 109, 113, 114, 126, 127, 128, 129, 130, 131, 144

Eastern: culture 41, 43; societies; 126; traditions 127
empathy 5, 21, 22, 55, 61, 62, 63, 90, 109, 122, 147, 152, 154
English 2, 16, 18, 25, 26, 28, 60, 66, 73, 75, 93, 98, 104, 108, 109, 111, 113, 121, 127, 140, 141, 152, 153

ethnic 3, 6, 12, 14, 15, 16, 18, 25, 27, 29, 31, 45, 55, 61, 63, 66, 76, 79, 107, 112, 152, 153
ethnicity 1, 2, 3, 14, 19, 26, 28, 31, 48, 49, 55, 61, 63, 70, 77, 79, 114, 121, 123, 136

Filipino 5, 75, 77, 83, 87, 90

Geisha 2, 27, 34, 36, 37
Great Round theory 41, 42, 54

HUMBLE model 65, 73, *see also* cultural humility

identity: 2, 4, 9 10, 12, 14, 17, 19, 22, 25, 26, 27, 29, 41, 44, 46, 51, 52, 54, 56, 57, 59, 61, 62, 65, 67, 75, 77, 85, 87, 90, 93, 97, 108, 115, 119, 121, 125, 128, 129, 134; development 14; negotiation 47, 48; racial and ethnic 15, 25, 53; struggle 12, 27, 60
immigrant 1, 4, 15, 18, 21, 25, 41, 46, 47, 49, 50, 51, 53, 55, 63, 83, 84, 89, 91, 96, 97, 98, 124
India(n) 3, 4, 5, 9, 10, 11, 12, 14, 15, 16, 17, 18, 19, 22, 41, 43, 49, 52, 65, 66, 67, 68, 69, 72, 73, 76, 89
intercultural 5, 121
intracultural 5, 121, 123, 125, 129, 131, 135

Japan(ese) 1, 2, 3, 4, 6, 7, 25, 27, 28, 29, 30, 31, 37, 38, 55, 59, 60, 61, 89, 93, 121, 124, 125, 129, 130, 131, 133, 134, 137, 139, 140, 141, 142, 143, 144, 147, 148, 151, 152, 153
Jung, C. 42, 43

Kimono 1, 2, 27, 36, 37
Korean 2, 59, 107, 108, 109, 110, 111, 114, 115, 118, 121, 151
Kramer, E. 66, 152

labeling 59, 60, 63

mandala 4, 41, 42, 43, 44, 45, 46, 72, 131
minority 90, 105, 121, 125, 142; clients 4, 5, 25; groups 60, 62, 63, 125 133; members 60, 62; membership 6, *see also* AATA;

model 60; race/ethnic 3, 45, 51, 55, 57; status 63; student 26, 76, 88; therapist 121, 122
multicultural(ism) 2, 3, 5, 16, 18, 20, 88, 105, 107, 151, 152, 154
mutual empathy 5, 55, 62

narrative(s) 3, 4, 5, 10, 11, 45, 50, 53, 55, 60, 63, 102, 104
narrative art therapy 5, 96, 100
narrative therapy 95, 97, 99, 100, 103
Native American 41, 44, 45, 49, 50, 51, 52, 54
non-White 3, 6, 26, 38, 152, 153

open art 30, 34
oppression 4, 11, 20, 21, 22, 45, 62, 104, 122, 125
Origami 31, 98, 135
othering 55, 56, 62, 63

painting(s) 12, 14, 58, 109, 110, 111, 112, 113, 114, 115, 116, 117, 118, 119, 120, 134, 135
Philippines 4, 75, 76, 77, 83, 84, 89
privilege 3, 10, 15, 18, 19, 20, 21, 38, 52, 60, 62, 105, 151

race 1, 3, 4, 5, 6, 20, 21, 27, 31, 48, 50, 51, 55, 105, 123, 135
race/ethnicity 2, 3, 14, 19, 26, 28, 31, 55, 63, 70, 121, 123
racism 6, 10, 15, 16, 19
racist 27, 31, 36

same race 5, 6, 123
self-awareness 5
self-esteem 49, 53, 78
self-knowledge 9, 53
self-perception 48
self-reflection 5, 9, 38, 48, 65, 93, 129, 135
South Korea(n) 2, 4, 27, 29, 30, 107, 111
stereotypes(d) 16, 17, 26, 29, 37, 61, 135, 153
stigma, stigmatized, stigmatizing 61, 63, 91, 95, 97, 100, 124, 140
Sumi(e) 31, 32, 33, 134, 135
supervisee 139, 143, 144, 145, 146, 147, 148

supervision 5, 6, 17, 48, 65, 67, 108, 125, 139, 142, 143, 144, 145, 146, 147, 148
supervisor(s) 2–3, 17, 27, 28, 36, 67, 68, 94, 95, 108, 139, 142, 143, 144, 147, 148

Taiwanese 5, 93, 151
The Red Book 42
therapeutic alliance 21, 109, 114
training 4, 6, 26, 27, 28, 55, 66, 68, 69, 70, 73, 94, 121, 126, 141, 143, 148, 151, 152, 153, 154
transference 9, 34
trauma(tic) 30, 52, 54, 86, 103

U.S. Census Bureau 89, 123
unconscious(ly) 42, 52, 55, 60, 61, 93, 133, 148

Western 12, 45, 52, 93, 125, 126; art therapy 6, 135; clothes 17, 41, 126; culture 43, 126; education 127; medication 30; supremacy 45; therapists 126, 127
White 5, 9, 11, 16, 18, 19, 20, 21, 27, 29, 38, 60, 83, 87, 89, 90, 104, 105, 122, 129, 134, 151, 152, 153; art therapist 2, 27 152; client 90; faculty 6; male 2, 18, 111; male supervisor 28; patient 3; profession 27, 127, 134, 135; professors 127; students 2, 6, 18; therapist 29, 122; woman 38
White Americans 2, 4, 5, 26, 27, 28, 29, 52, 60, 67, 108
White racial identity 15
White supremacy 10, 19, 21

For Product Safety Concerns and Information please contact our EU
representative GPSR@taylorandfrancis.com
Taylor & Francis Verlag GmbH, Kaufingerstraße 24, 80331 München, Germany